COMPACT *Research*

# Down Syndrome

**Diseases and Disorders**

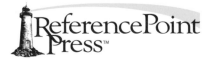

ReferencePoint
Press™

San Diego, CA

# Other books in the Compact Research series include:

## Current Issues

Abortion
Assisted Suicide
Biomedical Ethics
Civil Rights
Cloning
The Death Penalty
Energy Alternatives
Free Speech
Gay Rights
Health Care
Human Rights
Global Warming and
    Climate Change

Gun Control
Illegal Immigration
Islam
National Security
Nuclear Weapons and
    Security
Obesity
School Violence
Stem Cells
Terrorist Attacks
U.S. Border Control
Video Games
World Energy Crisis

## Diseases and Disorders

ADHD
Alzheimer's Disease
Anorexia
Autism
Bipolar Disorders
Hepatitis

HPV
Meningitis
Phobias
Sexually Transmitted
    Diseases

## Drugs

Alcohol
Club Drugs
Cocaine and Crack
Hallucinogens
Heroin
Inhalants
Marijuana

Methamphetamine
Nicotine and Tobacco
Performance-Enhancing
    Drugs
Prescription Drugs
Steroids

COMPACT *Research*

# Down Syndrome

by Peggy J. Parks

**Diseases and Disorders**

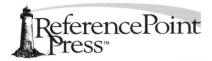

ReferencePoint
Press™

San Diego, CA

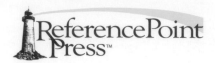

**For more information, contact:**
ReferencePoint Press, Inc.
PO Box 27779
San Diego, CA 92198
www.ReferencePointPress.com

Picture credits:
Maury Aaseng: 33–36, 49–51, 64–66, 80–82
AP Images: 14
Landov: 19

Parks, Peggy J., 1951–
    Down syndrome / by Peggy J. Parks.
      p. cm. — (Compact research)
    Includes bibliographical references and index.
    ISBN-13: 978-1-60152-065-4 (hardback)
    ISBN-10: 1-60152-065-4 (hardback)
    1. Down syndrome—Popular works. I. Title.
    RC571.P37 2008
    616.85'8842—dc22
                                                          2008036644

# Contents

# Foreword

**"Where is the knowledge we have lost in information?"**

—T.S. Eliot, "The Rock."

As modern civilization continues to evolve, its ability to create, store, distribute, and access information expands exponentially. The explosion of information from all media continues to increase at a phenomenal rate. By 2020 some experts predict the worldwide information base will double every 73 days. While access to diverse sources of information and perspectives is paramount to any democratic society, information alone cannot help people gain knowledge and understanding. Information must be organized and presented clearly and succinctly in order to be understood. The challenge in the digital age becomes not the creation of information, but how best to sort, organize, enhance, and present information.

ReferencePoint Press developed the *Compact Research* series with this challenge of the information age in mind. More than any other subject area today, researching current issues can yield vast, diverse, and unqualified information that can be intimidating and overwhelming for even the most advanced and motivated researcher. The *Compact Research* series offers a compact, relevant, intelligent, and conveniently organized collection of information covering a variety of current topics ranging from illegal immigration and methamphetamine to diseases such as anorexia and meningitis.

The series focuses on three types of information: objective single-author narratives, opinion-based primary source quotations, and facts and statistics. The clearly written objective narratives provide context and reliable background information. Primary source quotes are carefully selected and cited, exposing the reader to differing points of view. And facts and statistics sections aid the reader in evaluating perspectives. Presenting these key types of information creates a richer, more balanced learning experience.

For better understanding and convenience, the series enhances information by organizing it into narrower topics and adding design features that make it easy for a reader to identify desired content. For example, in *Compact Research: Illegal Immigration*, a chapter covering the economic impact of illegal immigration has an objective narrative explaining the various ways the economy is impacted, a balanced section of numerous primary source quotes on the topic, followed by facts and full-color illustrations to encourage evaluation of contrasting perspectives.

The ancient Roman philosopher Lucius Annaeus Seneca wrote, "It is quality rather than quantity that matters." More than just a collection of content, the *Compact Research* series is simply committed to creating, finding, organizing, and presenting the most relevant and appropriate amount of information on a current topic in a user-friendly style that invites, intrigues, and fosters understanding.

# Down Syndrome
# at a Glance

## What It Is

Down syndrome is a genetic disorder that includes varying combinations of birth defects, including some degree of mental retardation.

## Prevalence

An estimated 2 million people throughout the world have Down syndrome, with approximately 350,000 living in the United States.

## Cause

Down syndrome occurs because of abnormalities in chromosomes that usually develop before fertilization, or in very rare cases, after fertilization.

## Diagnosis

Because of certain physical features, Down syndrome can often be diagnosed as soon as a baby is born. The disorder is confirmed through a test known as a chromosomal karyotype.

## Health Issues

More than half of all babies born with Down syndrome have heart defects, from mild to severe. Other physical ailments may include vision problems, hearing loss, and a high susceptibility to infection and childhood leukemia, as well as early onset Alzheimer's disease.

## Life Expectancy

In the early twentieth century children with Down syndrome rarely lived past the age of nine. Today the average life expectancy is the mid-fifties, although some people live longer.

## Civil Rights

People with Down syndrome are protected against discrimination by the Individuals with Disabilities Education Act (IDEA) and the Americans with Disabilities Act (ADA).

## Ethical Issues

Prenatal testing can detect Down syndrome in a fetus with a high degree of accuracy. These tests are controversial because an estimated 90 percent of diagnosed cases result in abortion.

# Overview

In 1866 a British physician named John Langdon Down opened a residential psychiatric facility in England for people with a wide range of intellectual disabilities. Down was particularly interested in a group of patients who had varying degrees of mental retardation and shared similar physical characteristics. He began to study and photograph them, writing papers about his observations and giving presentations to other medical professionals. In 1887 Down published a book titled *On Some of the Mental Affections of Childhood and Youth*, in which he described these patients, whose physical features were so similar that those who were not even related looked like siblings. "They present characteristics so marked that when the members of this type are placed in proximity it is difficult to believe that they are not brothers and sisters," he wrote. "In fact their resemblance is infinitely greater to one another than to the members of their own families."[1] Down noted that the children he studied resembled those of Asian descent, particularly Mongolians, because of their slanted eyes. Their faces were flat and broad, their cheeks were round, and their lips were rather large. In addition, their noses and mouths were smaller than normal, and some had tongues that were so large and thick that it interfered with their speech. This condition came to be known as Down's syndrome (later changed to Down syndrome in the United States), although nearly a century passed before scientists knew what the disorder was and what caused it.

## What Is Down Syndrome?

Down Syndrome is a genetic disorder that includes varying combinations of birth defects. As Down noted, people who have Down syndrome have startlingly similar physical features. These often include an upward slant to the eyes; small ears that fold over at the top; round, slightly flattened faces; small mouths that make their tongues appear larger than normal; short limbs; and smaller-than-average stature. Although all have some degree of mental retardation, this can vary widely from person to person. As the National Down Syndrome Society (NDSS) states, "The effect [of mental retardation] is usually mild to moderate and is not indicative of the many strengths and talents that each individual possesses."[2] Physical characteristics may differ as well. Down syndrome is very apparent in some people's facial features, while in others the characteristics are barely recognizable. Nevertheless, there is no correlation between an individual's physical features and his or her degree of mental retardation.

> **Down noted that the children he studied resembled those of Asian descent . . . because of their slanted eyes.**

The personality traits of people with Down syndrome are often referred to as unique and refreshingly positive. Although no two are the same, those with Down syndrome are typically warm and cheerful by nature, as well as loving, gentle, patient, and tolerant. They are often described as having an attitude toward life that puts so-called "normal" people to shame. Martha Beck, whose teenage son Adam has Down syndrome, describes this attitude:

He zeroes in on anything there is to love about anyone and anything that crosses his path. He is a natural optimist, constantly finding things about which to feel enthusiastically pleased. I can't express how wonderfully it changes your daily life to spend it with someone who thinks this way. . . . Every day, his ready grin and easy gratitude teach me more about how to enjoy life than I learned during the twenty-plus years of my formal education.[3]

## Improved Lives

In the past, parents whose child was born with Down syndrome were strongly advised by health care professionals to put the infant into an institution. The babies were called derogatory names such as "Mongolian idiot" or "Mongoloid." It was erroneously believed that all Down syndrome children were so severely retarded that they had no chance whatsoever to live a high-quality life or to achieve any semblance of normalcy. Therapist Andrea Lack explains what parents of Down syndrome children typically heard: "The child would never walk, talk, read, or think; the child would not be able to relate to parents or family; and the child would remain a drain on the family financially and emotionally. In other words, having a child with Down syndrome was not accepted by society at large."[4]

> " There is no correlation between an individual's physical features and his or her degree of mental retardation. "

Without any sort of quality medical attention, therapy, stimulation, or opportunities to develop, children who were born with Down syndrome in the early 1900s rarely lived past the age of 9. In 1983 the average life expectancy was still only 25 years. Today, people with Down syndrome typically live until their mid-fifties, and many live longer than that. On January 26, 2009, Barbara Kendall, who was born with Down syndrome, celebrated her seventy-fifth birthday. She is believed to be the oldest woman in the United States with Down syndrome. "When she was born, they told her mother maybe she might live to be 32, 35; that would be it," says Kendall's stepsister and caregiver. "And here she is going strong."[5] Like most parents at the time of Kendall's birth, her mother was advised by doctors to place the baby in an institution, but she refused. Today, Kendall lives an active, happy life. Each day she rides a bus to an adult day care center, and she enjoys playing bingo, bocce ball, bowling, and watching the television program *The Price Is Right*.

## What Causes Down Syndrome?

Scientists have been studying Down syndrome for decades, but much about the disorder is still baffling to them. They now know that it is caused by abnormalities in chromosomes, gene-carrying structures that are found in all the cells of the body. Each person normally has 23 pairs of chromosomes, for a total of 46. For reasons that are still unknown, something goes wrong before fertilization (or in rare cases, after), causing an egg or sperm cell to develop incorrectly. As a result, the cell contains extra genetic material in chromosome 21, so the fetus inherits 47 chromosomes rather than the normal 46. This is also known as trisomy 21 because people with Down syndrome have 3 number-21 chromosomes rather than 2 in all the cells of the body. Trisomy 21 is the most common form of Down syndrome. Two other types that are much rarer are mosaicism (or mosaic Down syndrome) and translocation Down syndrome, which are also caused by chromosomal abnormalities.

## Does Parental Age Increase the Risk of Down Syndrome?

An estimated 80 percent of Down syndrome babies are born to women under age 35 because, by far, younger women have the most babies. The risk of Down syndrome increases dramatically as a woman gets older, though. At age 20 the chance of a woman giving birth to a baby with Down syndrome is about 1 in 1,600—and by age 49, the likelihood has risen to 1 in 12.

In 2003 researchers from Columbia University published a study that focused not only on older mothers but fathers as well. In the June 2003 issue of the *Journal of Urology*, they write: "The influence of maternal age on Down syndrome is well established but little is known about the genetic consequences of advanced paternal age."[6] The researchers studied 3,419 cases of Down syndrome that were reported to the New York State Department of Public Health from 1983 to 1997. Over the

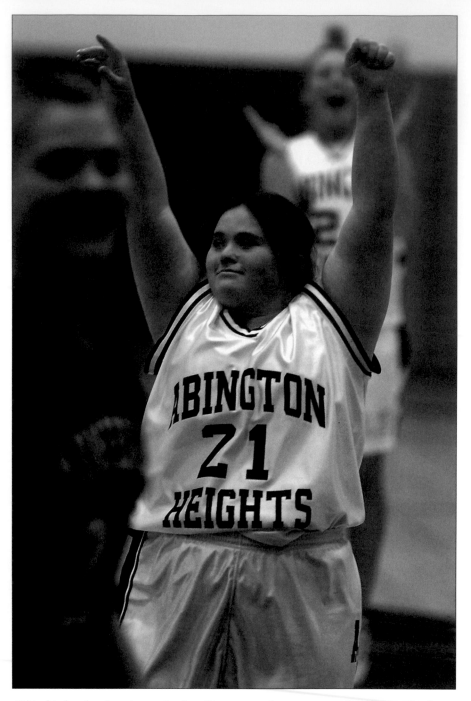

*This high school senior, who has Down syndrome, scores during her basketball game. People with Down syndrome now have many more opportunities to succeed than they ever did in the past.*

15-year period, they found no increase in the number of babies born to younger parents but a dramatic increase among parents who were older than 35: 111 percent for mothers and 60 percent for fathers. From this the researchers concluded that the highest risk of Down syndrome was advanced age in women, but men were a factor as well: "Advanced paternal age combined with maternal age significantly influences the incidence of Down syndrome. This effect may represent a paradigm for other genetic abnormalities in children of older fathers."[7]

## How Prevalent Is Down Syndrome?

Down syndrome is one of the most common genetic birth defects. According to the Centers for Disease Control and Prevention (CDC), Down syndrome occurs in about 1 out of every 740 live births in the United States, which is approximately 5,500 babies per year. An estimated 2 million people throughout the world have Down syndrome, with approximately 350,000 in the United States and 200,000 in Western Europe.

## How Down Syndrome Is Diagnosed

The symptoms of Down syndrome are usually obvious enough at the time of a baby's birth for physicians to diagnose it right away. Initially, the diagnosis is based on physical characteristics that are commonly seen in babies with Down syndrome. Mike Spellman is a physician, and when his son Anthony was born, Spellman noticed some telltale signs immediately. Anthony's face was slightly flattened, his eyes were slanted upward, and both of his palms had a single, deep crease, all of which are typical symptoms of Down syndrome. Other symptoms include white spots on the iris of the eye (known as "Brushfield spots"), a short neck, broad feet with short toes, and excessive space between the large and second toes.

Physical characteristics alone are not conclusive evidence that an infant has Down syndrome, however. Some of these features may also be found in

> " At age 20 the chance of a woman giving birth to a baby with Down syndrome is about 1 in 1,600—and by age 49, the likelihood has risen to 1 in 8. "

babies who are not affected by the disorder. If Down syndrome is suspected, it is usually confirmed by a test known as a chromosomal karyotype, which is a display of the chromosomes of a single cell. The karyotype involves "growing" cells from the baby's blood for about two weeks. Then a cell is stained with dye and visualized through a microscope just before cell division occurs, when the chromosomes are easiest to see. The karyotype provides a visual display of the chromosomes grouped according to size (from largest to smallest), number, and shape. This arrangement helps scientists identify specific chromosomal abnormalities with a high degree of accuracy.

## Related Health Issues

Many babies who are born with Down syndrome have a number of health problems. According to the March of Dimes, almost half of them have heart defects. Some of these defects are so minor that they heal themselves, while others may require surgery to correct. Anthony Spellman, for example, was born with a tiny hole between the two upper chambers of his heart, but it was not a life-threatening condition. The slight defect was expected to close naturally and heal on its own without surgery.

The extra genetic material in the chromosomes of Down syndrome children can also cause other physical ailments, such as vision problems, hearing loss, and a high susceptibility to infection. Children with Down syndrome are also at least 10 times more likely than those without it to develop leukemia, which is a cancer of the blood. Sarah Hanson, who was born with Down syndrome, was stricken with acute lymphocytic leukemia when she was a toddler. After treatment she went into remission, but her health problems did not stop there. Sarah also has a heart defect, as well as hydrocephalus, which is excessive fluid within the brain. In addition, at the age of 20 months Sarah suffered a series of strokes that left her a quadriplegic. When her cousin Emily received a school assignment to write a paragraph about a Christmas wish, she wrote the following:

> " Children with Down syndrome are also at least 10 times as likely as those without it to develop leukemia, which is a cancer of the blood. "

If I could give one wish to someone it would be my cousin Sarah. I wish that doctors could find all of the cures for Sarah's many diseases. One reason I would wish for this is so she wouldn't have to go to the hospital. . . . Sarah has multiple diseases and disabilities. I wish that I could find a cure for her leukemia also! . . . Sarah has a lot of complications and that is why I wished doctors could find a cure for them!"[8]

## The Importance of Early Intervention

Children with Down syndrome were once believed to be so mentally impaired that they were not teachable, but that is now known to be completely inaccurate. It has been proven that the earlier a child becomes involved with physical therapy and schooling, the more progress he or she can make—and many make astounding progress. According to the NDSS, programs are often individualized to meet the specific needs of each child and are designed to help infants and children reach growth milestones such as motor skills (holding and reaching for objects), language, social development, and self-help skills. Such early intervention programs should begin shortly after birth and continue until the child reaches the age of three. The NDSS explains how beneficial such programs are:

> Early intervention, research and case histories have shown that children with Down syndrome have a far greater potential for learning and for functioning as contributing members of society than it was believed to be possible even 10 to 15 years ago. . . . Optimistic, yet realistic, expectations plus the ability to recognize and reinforce the smallest increments of progress are the attitudes that are most likely to have a positive effect on development. In this way, early interventions succeed in maximizing achievement.[9]

## Civil Rights for the Disabled

Prior to the 1970s, people with Down syndrome faced discrimination on a daily basis. Children who had the disorder, for instance, could legally be refused admission to public schools. According to the U.S. Office of Special Education Programs, in 1970 schools in the United States "educated only one in five children with disabilities, and many states had laws excluding certain students, including children who were deaf, blind, emotionally disturbed, or mentally retarded."[10] That changed in 1975 when Public Law 94-142, the Education of All Handicapped Children Act, later named the Individuals with Disabilities Education Act (IDEA), was passed by Congress. The law mandates free, appropriate public education for children with disabilities in every state and locality across the country. Because of this legislation, the majority of children with Down syndrome now attend their neighborhood schools and are in regular classrooms.

> No cure for Down syndrome exists, nor is it possible to correct it before an infant is born, as with some other genetic disorders.

Another landmark piece of legislation for people with Down syndrome was the Americans with Disabilities Act (ADA), which was signed into law in 1990. In its statement for support of the law, Congress wrote that "historically, society has tended to isolate and segregate individuals with disabilities, and, despite some improvements, such forms of discrimination against individuals with disabilities continue to be a serious and pervasive social problem."[11] Prior to passage of the ADA, legislation was already in place to protect people from discrimination on the basis of race, color, sex, national origin, religion, or age, and the ADA extended that same protection to people with disabilities. They could no longer be discriminated against in employment, public accommodations, transportation, and services provided by state and local governments.

## What Are the Ethical Issues of Down Syndrome?

Because the risk of bearing a child with Down syndrome increases as women get older, those who are over age 35 are routinely advised to undergo prenatal testing in order to assess the risk of the disorder in the fetus. This is often a test known as amniocentesis, which involves the surgical insertion of a hollow needle through the abdominal wall and into the uterus. A sample of amniotic fluid, containing cells shed by the fetus, is extracted and sent to a laboratory for analysis. Another test is known as chorionic villus sampling (CVS), in which a tiny amount of tissue is extracted from the fetus and tested for the presence of extra genetic material on chromosome 21.

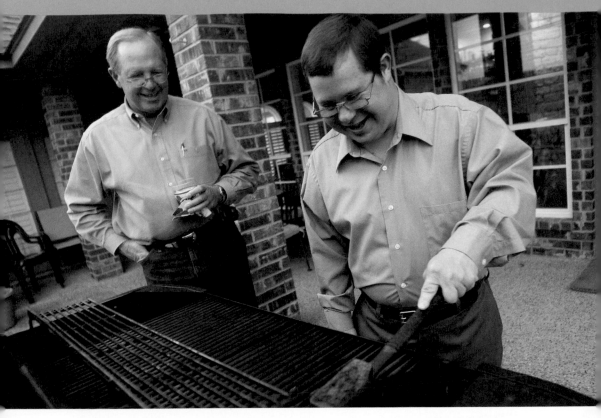

*This young man, who has Down syndrome, prepares the grill for a family barbeque. He enjoys spending time with his family but also has an independent life. In the past, parents whose child was born with Down syndrome were strongly advised by health care professionals to put the infant into an institution for his or her entire life.*

If prenatal test results are positive for Down syndrome, the parents can make a decision whether to continue with the pregnancy or terminate it. Such tests have long been highly controversial because an estimated 80 to 90 percent of prenatal diagnoses for Down syndrome result in abortions. According to Valerie Karr, who specializes in the rights of people with disabilities, more than 70 percent of pregnant women undergo prenatal screening. Karr also cites recent statistics showing that 92 percent of fetuses diagnosed with Down syndrome are now aborted. "Such abortions raise painful questions normally relegated to the religious or philosophical spheres," she writes. "Do we want only 'perfect' children? Does society value 'normal' people more than those with disabilities? Is the unalienable equality inherent in all humans a fraud?"[12]

## Will Research Someday Prevent Down Syndrome?

No cure for Down syndrome exists, nor is it possible to correct it before an infant is born, as with some other genetic disorders. Research continues to progress, however, and offers great hope for the future. For instance, a grant from the March of Dimes has helped to finance research into why errors of chromosome division occur, in the hope that this can lead to prevention. Researchers at the University of Colorado at Denver have performed experiments that could potentially result in therapies to increase the learning capacity of children and adults with Down syndrome. Studies with mice, which target the complex genetic factors involved in Down syndrome, are helping scientists learn more about what the proteins on chromosome 21 do and how they behave. This could potentially result in the ability to normalize chromosomal function, as researcher Wayne Silverman writes, "either by correcting imbalances or compensating for their presence. Key studies can literally be impossible to do in people for reasons that are self-evident. . . . No serious person would ever suggest that we manipulate people's genes just to explore the consequences. However, these types of studies can be done in animal 'models.'"[13]

Many people, however, argue that prevention methods or cures should not be pursued because people with Down syndrome are just as valuable to society as those who are not affected by it. If a cure is found, a time may eventually come when an entire class of people has been eliminated. As law professor Elizabeth Schiltz, who has a son with Down syndrome, explains: "People with Down syndrome wear their vulnerability on their faces. They are a visible reminder that the image of God reflected in humanity includes people of all sorts of intellectual capacities. It would be an impoverished society indeed that succeeded in eliminating such powerful teachers of both humanity and divinity."[14]

## Down Syndrome in the Future

Down syndrome is certainly much better understood today than it was when John Langdon Down identified it in the 1800s. Over the years scientists have learned what Down syndrome is and what causes it, although they still do not know why the various chromosomal disorders occur. With continued research, they may eventually gain the knowledge that allows them to prevent or cure Down syndrome. Whether such progress would be a triumph or a tragedy is a matter of personal opinion—and a controversial issue.

# What Is Down Syndrome?

> **Down syndrome is the most frequent genetic cause of mild to moderate mental retardation and associated medical problems and occurs . . . in all races and economic groups.**
>
> —James N. Parker and Philip M. Parker, eds., *The Official Parents' Sourcebook on Down Syndrome.*

> **The most important fact to know about individuals with Down syndrome is that they are more like others than they are different.**
>
> —National Association for Down Syndrome, "Facts About Down Syndrome."

Of all the diseases and disorders that exist, Down syndrome has historically been one of the least understood. As recently as 35 years ago, whenever a baby was diagnosed with Down syndrome, doctors assumed that parents would not want to care for their child and would immediately place him or her in an institution. This was the experience of syndicated columnist George Will, whose oldest son was born with Down syndrome in 1972. A geneticist at the hospital spoke with Will and his wife after the birth and asked if they intended to take their son home, to which they replied that "taking a baby home seemed like the thing to do." He explains: "Jon was born at the end of the era in which institutionalization of the retarded was considered morally acceptable, but in what was still an era of gross ignorance: In the first year of Jon's life, a network-television hospital drama featured a doctor telling parents of a Down syndrome newborn that their child would probably never be toilet-trained."[15] Emily Perl Kingsley, a writer for *Sesame Street*, also encountered this sort of attitude when her son Jason was born in June 1974. He was diagnosed with Down syndrome when he was just a few hours old. Kingsley and her husband were told by the doctor that their son would be mentally retarded and would never sit, stand, walk, or talk, nor would he ever be able to read or write or even have meaningful thoughts or ideas. The doctor strongly recommended that the Kingsleys place Jason in an institution right away, and even advised them to tell their friends and family that the baby died in childbirth. They were appalled at such a suggestion and vowed to give their son every opportunity to grow, learn, and thrive. Today, Jason is living on his own, working, and thoroughly enjoying life.

## Improved Health

The life expectancy for children who are born with Down syndrome has improved dramatically since the early twentieth century. A major reason is that so many of their accompanying physical problems can now be treated. Heart defects, for instance, occur in about 50 percent of babies born with Down syndrome. In the past these children were almost always doomed to die. Today, however, mild heart problems can often be treated with medications, while more serious defects can be repaired with surgery. Also, an estimated 10 percent of babies born with Down syndrome have stomach problems, or intestinal blockages that prevent them from digesting food properly. As with heart defects, these disorders can often be surgically corrected.

> **The doctor strongly recommended that the Kingsleys place Jason in an institution right away, and even advised them to tell their friends and family that the baby died in childbirth.**

For years it was widely believed that children with Down syndrome did not respond like normal children because they were severely retarded. It was later discovered, however, that the real problem was hearing deficiencies, which affected their ability to learn. It is now known that about 75 percent of children with Down syndrome have some sort of hearing loss, which is often caused by a buildup of fluid or mucus in the middle ear. For children with Down syndrome, the combination of even slight mental retardation with hearing loss can have a significant impact upon their ability to learn and communicate. Susan Snashall of St. George's University of London explains:

> People with intellectual impairment often have difficulty processing speech, especially in noise, and in locating the source of a sound. A mild hearing loss will make these tasks even more difficult. People with Down's syndrome are unlikely to complain of hearing impairment and it is necessary for hearing loss and middle ear disease to be detected by screening procedures if remedial action is not to be delayed.[16]

In addition to hearing defects, children born with Down syndrome often suffer from vision problems such as crossed eyes (a disorder known as esotropia) and near- or far-sightedness. In most cases wearing eyeglasses will correct these deficiencies. Cataracts, which interfere with vision by causing the lens of the eyes to become cloudy, are rare in children but common among those who have Down syndrome. According to the Children's Hospital in Boston, glasses may help in some cases, but surgical removal of cataracts is most often recommended in order to restore a child's vision.

## Benefits of Physical Therapy

Children who have Down syndrome tend to have a variety of problems with their muscles. For instance, they typically have poor muscle tone and extremely flexible joints, which cause their arms and legs to be "floppy." Because of that, when they try to sit up, crawl, or roll over, they adjust their movements to compensate for these deficiencies, and this can place undue stress on their joints. Physical therapy can help children learn proper movement techniques and overcome muscle deficiencies. Contrary to what is often believed, the goal of physical therapy is not to speed up the rate at which a child with Down syndrome reaches developmental milestones such as standing or walking. As the mother of a young boy with Down syndrome explains:

> The goal of physical therapy in Down Syndrome is to help the child learn to move his body in *appropriate ways*.

For example, hypotonia [low muscle tone] in a child with Down Syndrome may cause him to walk in a way that is not posturally correct. This is called compensation. Without physical therapy many, if not most, children who have Down Syndrome will adjust their movements to compensate for their low muscle tone. This can lead to problems, such as pain, in the future. So the goal of physical therapy is to teach proper physical movement.[17]

One particularly common trait in children with Down syndrome is that they learn to walk with their feet wide apart and turned out and their knees stiff. Physical therapists teach them to stand properly, with their feet positioned under the hips and pointing straight ahead and with their knees slightly bent. This helps their muscles develop properly and reduces the risk of overtaxing the muscles.

## Overcoming Mental Impairment

Unlike years ago when it was assumed that everyone with Down syndrome was severely retarded, it is now known that the degree of mental retardation varies widely from person to person. Most children born with Down syndrome have only mild to moderate mental impairment. With therapy and education, as well as love and encouragement from their families, they can make remarkable progress, often far beyond what is expected of them. Donald and Jeanne Bakely's daughter Beth was born with Down syndrome, and they enrolled her in an infant development center when she was just one month old. Beth attended classes at the center several times a week for

> " Children who have Down syndrome tend to have a variety of problems with their muscles. "

the next 5 years. Therapists worked with her on muscle development and balance, helped develop her cognitive skills, and helped her learn to speak clearly. By the time she was 5 years old, Beth was performing at a typical 5-year-old's level. When it was time for her to enter kindergarten, her parents were not sure if she would be able to attend a regular public school or if she would need special education. They met with school officials and expressed their concern. They were surprised and delighted at the response they received:

> We asked, "What about the Down Syndrome?" They said, "Look, we have kids in kindergarten—and all levels here—who don't speak English. We have kids whose parents never went to kindergarten, we have kids who never get breakfast, and are so hungry when they come to school, that they can't concentrate on what the teacher says, they can only think of their hunger. Beth's Down Syndrome seems to be a minor problem in light of some of these others. If she's doing 5-year-old stuff, we will put her in with the 5-year-olds. If she can't handle something, we'll deal with that—get her help, or try another approach. O.K.?"[18]

Beth entered kindergarten, and not only was she mainstreamed throughout all her school years, she continued to perform at her grade level. In 1994 she graduated from high school, and in 2001 she graduated from junior college with a certificate in recreational therapy. Bakely credits all the people who helped him and his wife enable his daughter to overcome the obstacles of Down syndrome and reach her full potential. "We don't know where life will take Beth," he writes, "but we know that the possibilities for her have been vastly stretched. There are hundreds of tasks, jobs, professions opened to her that there would not have been if it hadn't been for the schools, professionals, friends, and myriad helpers who went out of their way to train her and to slam doors open for her."[19]

> " Deegan is believed to be only one of two people in the United States with Down syndrome who sky-dives, and on June 11, 2008, he made his tenth jump. "

Casey Deegan is another real-life Down syndrome success story. His mental impairment is more severe than Beth Bakely's: At the age of 32 Deegan reads at a 5-year-old level, and he still talks about playing professional baseball for the Chicago White Sox when he grows up. Yet his life is full, active, and happy. He participates in the Special Olympics and has competed in track, softball, swimming, and weight lifting. Another of his favorite activities is skydiving. Deegan is believed to be only one of two people in the United States with Down syndrome who skydives, and on June 11, 2008, he made his tenth jump.

## Premature Aging

Because of all the progress that has been made in correcting physical and cognitive problems associated with Down syndrome, people who have it are living longer than ever before. That is good news, but it also presents some challenges because those with Down syndrome age an estimated 20 to 30 years ahead of people of the same age who are not afflicted with the disorder. This premature aging often leads to physical ailments that are typically experienced by elderly people, as neurologist Joseph R. Carcione explains:

> People with Down syndrome may experience health problems as they age that are similar to those experienced by older persons in the general population. The presence of extra genetic material found among persons with Down syndrome may lead to abnormalities in the immune system and a higher susceptibility to certain illnesses, such as Alzheimer's, leukemia, seizures, cataracts, breathing problems and heart conditions.[20]

> **Those with Down syndrome age an estimated 20 to 30 years ahead of people of the same age who are not afflicted with the disorder.**

Alzheimer's disease, which causes rapid, severe deterioration of the brain, is especially common among people with Down syndrome. It results in serious memory impairment and loss of bodily functions, and complications from it (such as pneumonia or infection) always lead to death. Alzheimer's most often affects older adults and is extremely rare in people who are younger than 65. But among many who have Down syndrome, symptoms show up years earlier. Maryann Slattery, whose mother died of Alzheimer's at the age of 80, has a 45-year-old sister with Down syndrome who is suffering from Alzheimer's disease. The once happy, bubbly, social woman is now quiet and withdrawn, and she looks and acts much older than her actual age. "You just see a little bit of her dying all the time," says Slattery. "With Alzheimer's, it's not just the person who has it. It's the family."[21]

## Challenges and Progress

Life for people with Down syndrome, and their families, is not always easy, and they face challenges every day. Yet opportunities abound today that were nonexistent in the past. No longer are Down syndrome babies written off as hopelessly retarded; instead, they are enrolled in special programs at an early age that help improve their cognitive skills and ability to communicate as well as overcome their physical challenges. Children often make such amazing progress that they graduate from high school and go on to college. Although people with Down syndrome have their differences, they have the same goals and dreams as those who do not have it, and all they want is to live happy, fulfilling lives. Now, more than ever before, this has become a reality for many of them. As Eunice Kennedy Shriver writes: "Fifty years ago children with Down syndrome were routinely excluded from public schools, could not play on playgrounds or prepare for jobs. Since then, however, they have made enormous contributions to our society, demonstrating a cardinal rule of life in America: With hard work you can accomplish what you dream."[22]

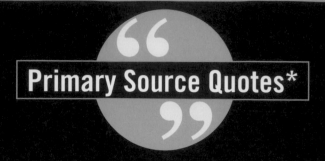

# Primary Source Quotes*

# What Is Down Syndrome?

❝No matter the gifts that arrive with a child who is something other than what you expected, and no matter how enthusiastically you embrace those gifts, there is still a loss to grieve, a loss of the child you thought you were going to have. It's an ache that, frankly, I don't know will ever go away.❞

—Karen Murphy, "Arthur Miller's Hidden Son: Dealing with Kids with Disabilities," StrollerDerby, August 23, 2007. www.babble.com.

Murphy is a writer who has a son with Down syndrome.

❝Penny is 27 months old. . . . She uses spoken and signed words to tell me what she did at school today, and the names of her friends, and what she would like for her afternoon snack. Penny loves music. She's learning her shapes and colors. She gives lots of hugs. . . . She is my daughter. She is my daughter with Down syndrome.❞

—Amy Julia Becker, "Down Syndrome Is a Part of Who My Daughter Is," *Philadelphia Inquirer*, July 20, 2008. www.philly.com.

Becker is a student at Princeton Theological Seminary.

* Editor's Note: While the definition of a primary source can be narrowly or broadly defined, for the purposes of Compact Research, a primary source consists of: 1) results of original research presented by an organization or researcher; 2) eyewitness accounts of events, personal experience, or work experience; 3) first-person editorials offering pundits' opinions; 4) government officials presenting political plans and/or policies; 5) representatives of organizations presenting testimony or policy.

**❝ It is mysterious as to why this is the case, but it turns out that everyone with Down syndrome—everyone— shows the full-blown pathology of Alzheimer's disease by age 40. ❞**

—William Mobley, "Dr. William Mobley on Down Syndrome and Upcoming Fundraiser," *LAist*, August 26, 2007. www.laist.com.

Mobley is professor and chair of the Department of Neurology and Neurological Sciences at Stanford University, as well as codirector of the Center for Research and Treatment of Down Syndrome at Stanford.

**❝ Every single day, he faces a world in which he has to work very hard to live an ordinary life—harder than we have ever had to—and he is prepared to put that effort in, every single day. We think he's a bit of a hero. He does more than just live—he lights up our world. ❞**

—Jill O'Connor, "My Son Has Down Syndrome," NineMSN Health, 2004. http://health.ninemsn.com.au.

O'Connor is the information services manager for Down Syndrome New South Wales in Australia.

**❝ People with Down syndrome have goals and dreams. They want to be heard and given the same respect as everyone else. Individuals with Down syndrome are thinking and feeling people, and they want to be treated as such. They want the same quality of life as everyone else. ❞**

—Mile High Down Syndrome Association (MHDSA), "Facts About Down Syndrome." www.mhdsa.org.

The MHDSA is an organization in Denver, Colorado, that provides education, resources, and support to families of children and adults with Down syndrome.

66 There is still a stigma attached to children born with Down syndrome. Mothers recall hearing nurses whispering about their children or how they themselves cried for days. 99

—Keith O'Brien, "He Uses Thursdays to Bust Stereotypes," *Boston Globe*, July 11, 2005. www.boston.com.

O'Brien is a staff writer for the *Boston Globe* and a regular contributor to other publications, including the *Boston Globe Sunday Magazine*, and several National Public Radio shows.

66 Sam has taught us much: live life to the fullest, smile as much as you can, laugh from your soul, never take for granted the little things in life and each and every day give someone a hug and let them know you love them. 99

—Sue Mayer, "Sam's Journey to 'Reach for the Stars,'" *Exceptional Parent*, February 2007.

Mayer is a woman from Wisconsin whose son has Down syndrome.

66 To Max, life is one big adventure: he chooses to see his cup as half full, positively overflowing, never half empty. Perhaps we could all learn a lesson from that. 99

—Sandy Lewis, "My 15-Year-Old Son Has Down Syndrome—but He's Already a Hollywood Star," *Daily Mail*, May 15, 2008. www.dailymail.co.uk.

Lewis is a woman from the United Kingdom whose teenaged son Max has Down syndrome.

66 The big surprise was that he was beautiful. I had been terrified of having a child I didn't want to look at. But Paddy has a wide smile, crinkly blue eyes and corn-coloured hair: he is adorable. 99

—Annie Rey, "I Half-Hoped That I Might Miscarry," *Guardian*, June 2, 2008. www.guardian.co.uk.

Rey is a woman from the United Kingdom whose son has Down syndrome.

**" Not only are children with Down Syndrome people too, they inspire a deep love and enthusiastic appreciation. "**

—Kathryn Jean Lopez, "Don't Be Down on Palin," *National Review*, July 30, 2008. http://article.nationalreview.com.

Lopez is a syndicated columnist and an editor for *National Review Online*.

**" Our children and young adults with Down syndrome . . . have dreams and goals just like every other human being, and they deserve the opportunity to realize their full potential. "**

—Suzanne Boudrot Shea, "Statement of Suzanne Boudrot Shea Before the Commission on the Future of Higher Education," March 20, 2006. www.ndsccenter.org.

Shea, who is president of the Massachusetts Down Syndrome Congress, has a young daughter with Down syndrome.

**" Even though people with Down syndrome may have some physical and mental features in common, symptoms of Down syndrome can range from mild to severe. "**

—National Institute of Child Health and Human Development (NICHD), "Down Syndrome," February 16, 2007. www.nichd.nih.gov.

The NICHD conducts and supports research on topics related to the health of children, adults, and families.

**" In addition to affecting physical appearance, the syndrome can cause hearing loss, heart malformations, hypertension, digestive problems and vision disorders. "**

—Susan J. Landers, "Down Syndrome Is the Target of Ambitious NIH Research Initiatives," *American Medical News*, February 25, 2008. www.ama-assn.org.

Landers covers public health, science, and related federal policy issues for *American Medical News*, a publication of the American Medical Association.

# Facts and Illustrations

## What Is Down Syndrome?

- According to the March of Dimes, an estimated **8 million children** (about 6 percent of total births worldwide) are born with Down syndrome or other serious birth defects.

- Down Syndrome Education International estimates that there are more than **2 million** people with Down syndrome worldwide.

- An estimated **350,000 people** with Down syndrome live in the United States.

- Trisomy 21 occurs in more than **90 percent** of Down syndrome cases.

- Once a baby is born with Down syndrome, he or she will always have **extra chromosomal material**.

- The life expectancy of people with Down syndrome has risen from less than 9 years in the early 1900s to the **mid-fifties**.

- Children with Down syndrome are 10 to 15 times more likely to develop **leukemia** than normal children.

- Children with Down syndrome have a **62 percent** higher incidence of pneumonia than those without the disorder.

- Approximately **50 percent** of babies born with Down syndrome have congenital heart disease.

# Physical Characteristics of Down Syndrome

Children with Down syndrome often have physical traits that can be identified by doctors at birth, and as they continue to develop certain features become more pronounced. This photograph shows some of the most common features.

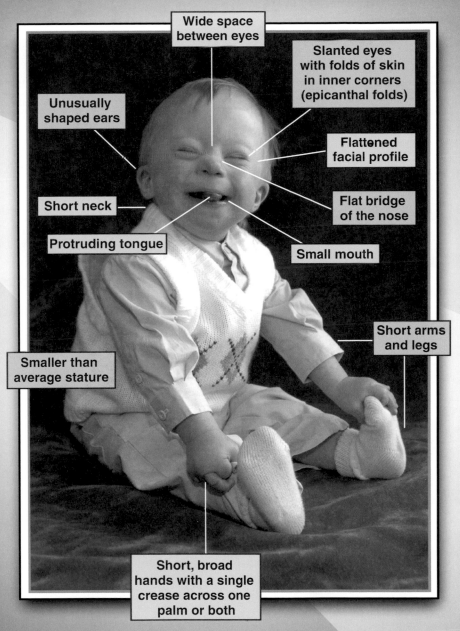

Wide space between eyes

Slanted eyes with folds of skin in inner corners (epicanthal folds)

Unusually shaped ears

Flattened facial profile

Short neck

Flat bridge of the nose

Protruding tongue

Small mouth

Short arms and legs

Smaller than average stature

Short, broad hands with a single crease across one palm or both

Source: National Dissemination Center for Children with Disabilities, "Down Syndrome," January 2004. http://old.nichcy.org.

## Medical Complications

Down syndrome is often accompanied by varying combinations of birth defects. This chart shows some of the most typical medical problems suffered by people who have the disorder.

| Disorder | Incidence |
|---|---|
| Mental retardation | > 95 percent |
| Growth retardation | > 95 percent |
| Vision disorders | > 60 percent |
| Hearing loss | 75 percent |
| Heart defects | 40 to 50 percent |
| Intestinal malformations | 12 percent |
| Epilepsy | 5 to 10 percent |
| Thyroid disorders | 5 percent |
| Leukemia | 1 percent |
| Early-onset Alzheimer's disease | Affects 75 percent by age 60 |
| Infertility | 99 percent in men; lack of ovulation in 30 percent in women |

Sources: Mahmoud Tarek, "The Baby with Down Syndrome," *Ain Shams Journal of Obstetrics and Gynecology*, September 2005. www.asjog.org; March of Dimes, "Down Syndrome," March 2007. www.marchofdimes.com.

- Research has shown that **66 to 89 percent** of children with Down syndrome have a hearing loss of greater than 15 to 20 decibels in at least one ear.

- The National Institute of Child Health and Human Development states that males with Down syndrome generally have a reduced sperm count and can **rarely father children**.

# The Most Common Birth Defects

According to the Centers for Disease Control and Prevention (CDC), birth defects occur in about 3 percent of all births in the United States, and are a leading cause of infant death and childhood disease. The CDC states that Down syndrome is one of the most common types of genetic defects; this graph shows how it compares with other types of congenital abnormalities.

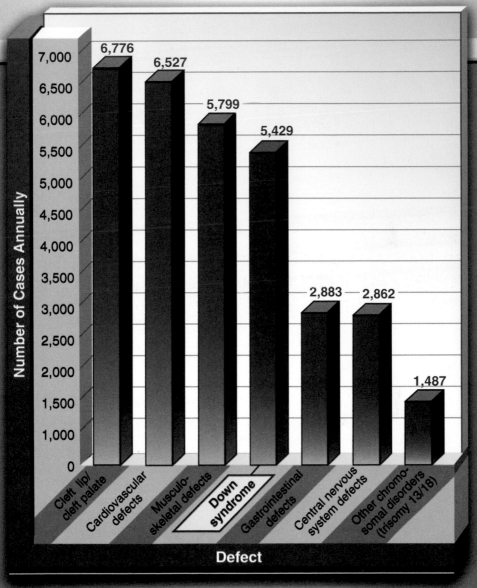

Number of Cases Annually

| Defect | Cases |
|---|---|
| Cleft lip/cleft palate | 6,776 |
| Cardiovascular defects | 6,527 |
| Musculoskeletal defects | 5,799 |
| Down syndrome | 5,429 |
| Gastrointestinal defects | 2,883 |
| Central nervous system defects | 2,862 |
| Other chromosomal disorders (trisomy 13/18) | 1,487 |

Defect

Source: Centers for Disease Control and Prevention, "National Estimates of and Racial and Ethnic Variations Among Selected Birth Defects," January 14, 2008. www.cdc.gov.

# The Importance of Chromosomes

Human bodies are made up of trillions of cells, and within the nucleus of each cell are long, threadlike structures called chromosomes. This illustration shows a normal cell structure and its associated chromosomes, genes, and strands of DNA.

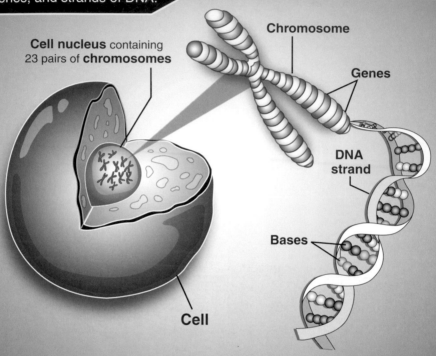

**Cell nucleus** containing 23 pairs of **chromosomes**

Chromosome

Genes

DNA strand

Bases

Cell

Sources: University of Utah Genetic Science Learning Center, "What Are Chromosomes?" 2008. http://learn.genetics. utah.edu; National Institute on Aging, "Alzheimer's Disease Genetics Fact Sheet," July 24, 2008. www.niah.nih.gov.

- Most females with Down syndrome have regular menstrual periods and are capable of becoming **pregnant**.

- According to the March of Dimes, a woman with Down syndrome has a **50-50 chance** of conceiving a child with Down syndrome.

# What Causes Down Syndrome?

> **A random event during the formation of reproductive cells or during very early development leads to Down syndrome. These events do not appear to be attributable to any behavioral activity of the parents or environmental factors.**
>
> —NIH Down Syndrome Working Group, "National Institutes of Health Research Plan on Down Syndrome."

> **What we do know is that no one is to blame. Nothing done before or during pregnancy can cause Down's syndrome. It occurs in all races, social classes and in all countries throughout the world. It can happen to anyone.**
>
> —Down's Syndrome Association, "Frequently Asked Questions."

In the years following John Langdon Down's identification of Down syndrome, scientists still struggled to find out what caused it. During the 1930s researchers stated that because the physical features of the disorder made it recognizable in people all over the world, it was undoubtedly some sort of genetic condition. Others theorized that advanced age in mothers played a role in the development of Down syndrome, which was later proved to be true. Some scientists correctly speculated that it was related to chromosomes, although no one could show definitive evidence of this theory. It was not until 1958 that Jerome Lejeune, a prominent French geneticist, confirmed that Down syndrome is a genetic disorder caused by chromosomal abnormalities. Scientists had developed a way for cells to be displayed on a microscopic slide so that chromosomes could be easily examined and counted, and Lejeune used this technique to analyze human cells. Peering through a powerful microscope, he could see that a normal human cell contained 46 chromosomes (23 pairs), while on a cell from one of his patients with Down syndrome he counted 47 chromosomes. Lejeune named the condition trisomy 21: *tri*, the Latin prefix for "three" and *somy*, which refers to a type of chromosome. Throughout the following years Lejeune became a well-known and outspoken advocate for humane care of people with Down syndrome. He was adamantly against prenatal testing for the disorder and was convinced that it would be possible in the future to correct chromosome abnormalities. He continued to pursue this research in an effort to discover why the abnormalities occurred. At the time of his death in 1994 he had still not found the answers he sought—and today, scientists still remain mystified about why these abnormalities happen.

> **Peering through a powerful microscope, [Lejeune] could see that a normal human cell contained 46 chromosomes (23 pairs), while on a cell from one of his patients with Down syndrome he counted 47.**

## Chromosomes and Trisomy 21

In order to understand how Down syndrome occurs, it is important to know what chromosomes are and the role they play in human development. When an egg and sperm are joined together at conception, this forms a fertilized egg known as a zygote (the earliest form of an embryo). Inside the zygote are chromosomes, which are long, thin, threadlike structures that are made up of proteins and deoxyribonucleic acid (DNA), the genetic "blueprint" of all living things. The National Human Genome Research Institute explains the significance of chromosomes: "The unique structure of chromosomes keeps DNA tightly wrapped around spool-like proteins, called histones. Without such packaging, DNA molecules would be too long to fit inside cells. For example, if all of the

DNA molecules in a single human cell were unwound from their histones and placed end-to-end, they would stretch 6 feet [1.8m]."[23] Unlike all the other cells of the body, each of which contains 46 chromosomes, an ovum and sperm each contains 23 chromosomes. During normal fertilization, a complete set of 46 chromosomes is passed to the zygote, half of which come from the mother and half from the father. A fertilized egg that will develop into a female contains chromosome pairs 1 through 22 and the XX pair (known as the sex chromosome), while a fertilized egg that will develop into a male contains pairs 1 through 22 and the XY pair. After the zygote has formed, it begins its developmental phase by dividing into 2 cells, then 4, then 8, then 16, and so on. During this process chromosomes also divide and replicate. If nothing goes wrong, every cell in the developing child's body will have the same number of chromosomes (with the exception of XX or XY chromosomes) that were originally contained in the fertilized egg: a total of 46.

For unknown reasons, an egg or sperm cell sometimes develops an extra chromosome 21. Thus, when fertilization occurs, the embryo will have 3 chromosomes 21 rather than the usual 2. This condition, which Lejeune named trisomy 21, occurs in more than 90 percent of Down syndrome cases. All cells in the bodies of children with trisomy 21 have 47 chromosomes instead of 46, with 3 copies of chromosome 21 in each cell.

## Translocation Down Syndrome

An estimated 3 to 4 percent of babies born with Down syndrome have a type that is known as translocation Down syndrome. As with trisomy 21, this is also the result of chromosomal abnormalities, but they occur in a different way. Either prior to or during conception, a section of chromosome 21 breaks off and "transfers its location," meaning it becomes stuck onto another chromosome in the egg or sperm cell, most commonly chromosome 14. In some cases the extra piece of chromosome 21 attaches itself to a normal pair of chromosomes 21. This occurred in an infant born to Christina Molin, a Swedish woman who lives in Austria. In May 2006 Molin's son Vince was diagnosed with translocation Down syndrome. When doctors showed her Vince's chromosomal chart, she could see an unusual phenomenon: His pair of twenty-first chromosomes had grown together, creating one chromosome that was larger than the average size, and the third twenty-first chromosome was sitting next to the newly formed one. She learned that when this sort of chromosomal abnormality occurs, there is a 99.5 percent likelihood "that it is just nature playing a trick on us, and this has nothing to do with inheritance."[24]

It is possible, however, for translocation Down syndrome to be inherited. In fact, it is the only form of the disorder that can be passed on from parent to child. The Mayo Clinic states that this occurs because either the mother or father is a "balanced" translocation carrier, meaning that in one of the parents, genetic material from chromosome 21 broke away and attached itself to a different chromosome. Thus, either the mother or the father has 45 chromosomes instead of the usual 46, and only one chromosome 21 rather than 2. The carrier will not have any characteristics of Down syndrome because he or she has no extra genetic material. The Mayo Clinic states that only about half of translocation Down syndrome cases are inherited. But according to the National Institute of Child Health and Human Development (NICHD), an infant who is born with translocation Down syndrome will be a carrier of the disorder and can potentially pass it on to any of his or her children who are born in the future.

> It is . . . possible for translocation Down syndrome to be inherited. In fact, it is the only form of the disorder that can be passed on from parent to child.

## Mosaicism

The rarest form of Down syndrome is mosaicism, which is also called mosaic Down syndrome or mosaic trisomy 21. Scientists are not exactly sure how or why mosaicism occurs, but they know that it occurs after fertilization rather than before and is caused by an error in cell division. The prevailing theory is that the zygote initially has 3 chromosomes 21, which would usually result in a baby with trisomy 21. But as the chromosomes are dividing and multiplying early in the embryo's development, some cells acquire extra genetic material while others do not. For example, the embryo may have 3 number 21 chromosomes in skin and blood cells, but the normal 2 chromosomes 21 in brain or bone marrow cells. For this reason, parents of children with mosaicism are sometimes told that their child has a "milder form" of Down syndrome. The National Down Syndrome Society describes the cells of these children as having a "mosaic" pattern, which the group compares to "the mosaic style of art in which a picture is made up of different colors of tiles."[25]

Because babies with mosaicism do not have an extra chromosome in all of their bodies' cells, symptoms of the disorder may not be evident at the time of birth. As a result, the children are often diagnosed later than those who have other forms of Down syndrome. Even if symptoms are present when a child is born, it can be difficult for physicians to accurately diagnose mosaicism. If the disorder is suspected, a sampling of the baby's cells are typically examined under a microscope. If the cells that are checked do not contain the extra chromosome, the diagnosis cannot be confirmed. This is what happened when Samantha Bell was born. At the time of her birth she only had slight symptoms of Down syndrome. As time went by, she seemed to be developing normally except for having some trouble with speech, which is a common trait among children with mosaicism. When Samantha was 3 years old, her doctor recommended that she have a chromosomal karyotype. The test confirmed that Samantha had mosaicism, but only about 16 percent of her body's cells contained the extra genetic material.

> Another characteristic of mosaicism is that many children who have the disorder lack the pronounced physical features of those who have trisomy 21.

Another characteristic of mosaicism is that many children who have the disorder lack the pronounced physical features of those who have trisomy 21. Claudia Vandervliet's daughter Shayenne was born with mosaicism in 1999, and when she was a toddler no one could tell that she had Down syndrome at all. Also, children with mosaicism often suffer from fewer cognitive difficulties than those with trisomy 21. Research has shown that these children often have a higher intelligence quotient (IQ) than those with trisomy 21, and they also typically reach developmental milestones earlier. By the time Shayenne was 13 months old, she was already starting to walk.

## Older Moms

Although women of any age can have a baby with Down syndrome, the risk increases with age, as the NICHD explains: "Researchers have established that the likelihood that a reproductive cell will contain an extra copy of chromosome 21 increases dramatically as a woman ages. Therefore, an older mother is more likely than a younger mother to have a baby with Down syndrome."[26] The frequency of a woman under 30 years old having a child with the disorder is 1 in 1,000, while at age 42 her chances have risen to 1 in 60. Scientists have long known that in most cases, the extra genetic material in chromosomes comes from the mother's egg rather than the father's sperm. One study that was published in the 1990s traced the extra chromosome to the mother's egg in 95 percent of the cases of Down syndrome, while only 5 percent were traced to the father's sperm. According to the Mayo Clinic, as a woman's eggs age, the likelihood that their chromosomes will divide improperly increases. Because women pass on the extra genetic material to an embryo so much more often than men, this helps explain why the risk is so much higher in older mothers.

> The frequency of a woman under 30 years old having a child with the disorder is 1 in 1,000, while at age 42 her chances have risen to 1 in 60.

Alaska governor, and the Republican vice-presidential nominee for the 2008 presidential election, Sarah Palin was aware of the risk when she became pregnant with her fifth child at the age of 44. Still, when she was 4 months along and prenatal testing showed that her baby had Down syndrome, she was somewhat shocked. Palin came to terms with the news, however, and began researching the disorder so she could prepare herself to do all that was necessary for her baby. On April 18, 2008, she gave birth to a son, Trig Paxson Van Palin. She and her husband were not unhappy that he had Down syndrome; instead, they believed that they had been blessed with a child who was special. She explains: "I'm looking at him right now, and I see perfection. Yeah, he has an extra chromosome. I keep thinking, in our world, what is normal and what is perfect?"[27]

## A Mysterious Disorder

Much progress has been made over the years as scientists have continued to study Down syndrome. They have identified three types of the disorder, and know that all are caused by various chromosomal abnormalities. They also know that the older a woman is, the greater her risk for giving birth to a child with the disorder. Yet with all that has been learned, Down syndrome is still puzzling in many ways. Why do chromosomal abnormalities occur? Why do they happen in some developing embryos and not others? Why do the physical symptoms and health problems vary so much from one child to the next? Why is only one form of Down syndrome hereditary, while the other two are not? And how can parents with no signs or symptoms pass it to their offspring? In the future, scientists may discover answers to those questions. For now, however, much about Down syndrome remains a mystery.

# Primary Source Quotes*

## What Causes Down Syndrome?

> 66 Today we can boldly predict that Down syndrome is not too complex to understand and it is not too difficult or too late to treat. 99

Down Syndrome Research and Treatment Foundation (DSRTF), "About Down Syndrome," 2007. www.dsrtf.org.

The DSRTF's focus is on biomedical research that will accelerate the development of treatments to significantly improve cognition for individuals with Down syndrome.

> 66 Scientists believe that Down syndrome is a disorder that is too complex and difficult to understand, let alone one for which effective treatments can be found. For this reason, the government invests little money in Down syndrome research. 99

—William C. Mobley and Craig C. Garner, "Message from the Directors," 2008. http://dsresearch.stanford.edu.

Mobley and Garner are codirectors of the Center for Research and Treatment of Down Syndrome at the Stanford School of Medicine.

Bracketed quotes indicate conflicting positions.

* Editor's Note: While the definition of a primary source can be narrowly or broadly defined, for the purposes of Compact Research, a primary source consists of: 1) results of original research presented by an organization or researcher; 2) eyewitness accounts of events, personal experience, or work experience; 3) first-person editorials offering pundits' opinions; 4) government officials presenting political plans and/or policies; 5) representatives of organizations presenting testimony or policy.

**&&** Circa 1920s, a diagnosis of Down syndrome was particularly heart crushing. Babies born with the condition often died during childhood. **&&**

—Society for Neuroscience, "Down Syndrome," *Brain Briefings*, April 2005. www.sfn.org.

The Society for Neuroscience is a membership organization of scientists and physicians who study the brain and nervous system.

........................................................................................................................................

**&&** Researchers have extensively studied the defects in chromosome 21 that cause Down syndrome. In 88% of the cases, the extra copy of chromosome 21 is derived from the mother. **&&**

—James N. Parker and Philip M. Parker, eds., *The Official Parents' Sourcebook on Down Syndrome*. San Diego: ICON, 2004.

James N. Parker is an author and lecturer, and Philip M. Parker is a university professor.

........................................................................................................................................

**&&** Down syndrome . . . is a genetic condition that affects about 1 in 800 babies, but it affects many more babies who are born to older women. **&&**

—Centers for Disease Control and Prevention (CDC), "Birth Defects: Frequently Asked Questions," July 18, 2007. www.cdc.gov.

The CDC is the federal agency charged with promoting health and quality of life by controlling disease, injury, and disability.

........................................................................................................................................

**&&** Most cases of Down syndrome aren't inherited. They're caused by a mistake in cell division during the development of the egg, sperm or embryo. **&&**

—Mayo Clinic, "Children's Health: Down Syndrome," April 6, 2007. www.mayoclinic.com.

Mayo Clinic is a world-renowned medical facility that is dedicated to the diagnosis and treatment of virtually every type of illness.

........................................................................................................................................

**❝When the fertilized egg contains extra material from chromosome 21, this results in Down syndrome.❞**

—National Institute of Child Health and Human Development (NICHD), "Facts About Down Syndrome," August 18, 2006. www.nichd.nih.gov.

The NICHD conducts and supports research on topics related to the health of children, adults, families, and populations.

**❝As far as we know, Down syndrome is not caused by any behavioral activity of the parents or environmental factors.❞**

—Arthur Schoenstadt, "Causes of Down Syndrome," eMedTV, July 7, 2008. http://down-syndrome.emedtv.com.

Schoenstadt is a physician who oversees the content development and review process for eMedTV.

**❝Although there is no conclusive evidence that specific environmental factors cause chromosome abnormalities, it is still a possibility that the environment may play a role in the occurrence of genetic errors.❞**

—Genetics Home Reference, "Can Changes in the Number of Chromosomes Affect Health and Development?" July 25, 2008. http://ghr.nlm.nih.gov.

Genetics Home Reference, a product of the National Library of Medicine, provides information about genetic conditions and the genes or chromosomes related to those conditions.

❝Many studies have analyzed the relationship between prenatal exposure to [oral contraceptives] and Down syndrome; the results are conflicting.❞

—Lev D. Kandinov, "Periconceptual Exposure to Oral Contraceptives and Risk for Down Syndrome," *Medscape Today*, 2005. www.medscape.com.

Kandinov is a physician at the Albert Einstein College of Medicine/Montefiore Medical Center in Bronx, New York.

❝Normally, we inherit 23 chromosomes from our mother and 23 chromosomes from our father (for a total of 46). Babies with Down syndrome inherit an extra copy of chromosome 21 leading to 3 copies (one from Mom, one from Dad, plus one extra). We call this *Trisomy 21.*❞

—Kyla Boyse, "Your Child: Down Syndrome (Trisomy 21)," University of Michigan Health System, January 2007. www.med.umich.edu.

Boyse is a registered nurse with the University of Michigan Health System.

# What Causes Down Syndrome?

- When a fertilized egg contains **extra genetic material** on chromosome 21, this results in Down syndrome.

- Trisomy 21 is caused by **chromosomal abnormalities** that occur before fertilization.

- Translocation Down syndrome occurs either before or during conception, while **mosaicism** occurs after fertilization.

- Some studies suggest that women who have certain **variant genes** that affect how their bodies metabolize the B vitamin folic acid may be at increased risk for having a baby with Down syndrome.

- Women under age 30 have less than a **1 in 1,000** chance of having a baby with Down syndrome; at the age of 49, the likelihood increases to **1 in 12**.

- Some studies have shown that a **father's age** also has an impact on whether a child will develop Down syndrome.

- Although older women have a much higher risk of having babies with Down syndrome, they account for only about **9 percent** of all live births and **25 percent** of Down syndrome births because younger women have more babies.

## Testing for Down Syndrome

Down syndrome can often be diagnosed when an infant is born because physical symptoms (such as slanted eyes, a flattened facial profile, and a single crease across one or both palms) are obvious, but a postnatal test known as a karyotype is used to confirm the diagnosis. This illustration shows the extra copy of chromosome 21 that children born with trisomy 21, the most common type of Down syndrome, have in every cell of their bodies.

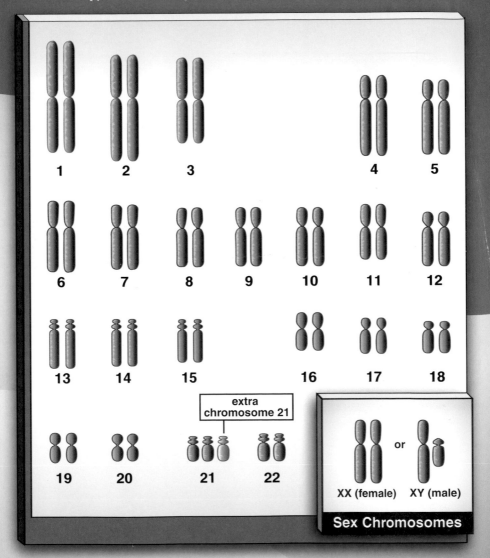

extra chromosome 21

XX (female)    XY (male)

**Sex Chromosomes**

Source: U.S. National Library of Medicine, "Genetics Home Reference Handbook," August 8, 2008. http://ghr.nlm.gov.

# When Chromosomes Go Awry

There are three types of Down syndrome: trisomy 21, which occurs in an estimated 90 percent or all cases; translocation Down syndrome; and mosaicism, which is the rarest type. All are caused by extra genetic material on chromosome 21, although the abnormalities occur in different ways. This illustration shows the development of an embryo with trisomy 21 compared with one with mosaicism.

## Trisomy 21

When fertilization occurs, the embryo will have 47 chromosomes, including 3 copies of chromosome 21.

The fertilized egg begins to divide, making more cells.

As cell division continues, the embryo will have 3 copies of chromosome 21 in every cell.

## Mosaicisim

When fertilization occurs, the embryo will have 47 chromosomes, including 3 copies of chromosome 21.

The fertilized egg begins to divide, making more cells.

As cell division continues, some cells acquire extra genetic material, while others do not

Both cell types continue to divide, making more cells; some have 3 chromosomes 21, other have 2

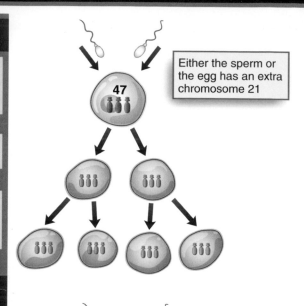

Either the sperm or the egg has an extra chromosome 21

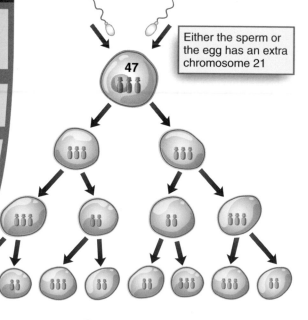

Either the sperm or the egg has an extra chromosome 21

Source: National Institute of Child Health and Human Development, "Facts About Down Syndrome," August 15, 2008. www.nichd.nih.gov.

## Chance of Down Syndrome Increases with Mother's Age

The number of infants born with Down syndrome is much higher among women under the age of 35 because they have the most babies. But the risk of having a child with the disorder increases exponentially as a woman ages.

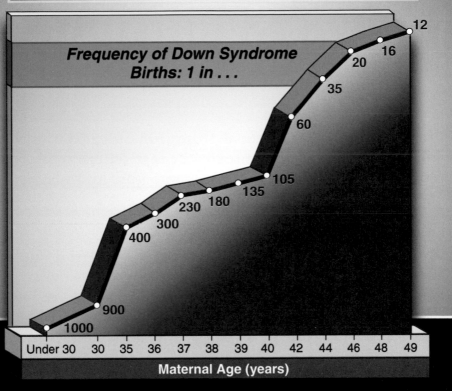

**Frequency of Down Syndrome Births: 1 in . . .**

12
16
20
35
60
105
135
180
230
300
400
900
1000

Maternal Age (years)

Under 30 · 30 · 35 · 36 · 37 · 38 · 39 · 40 · 42 · 44 · 46 · 48 · 49

Source: National Institute of Child Health and Human Development, "Facts About Down Syndrome," August 15, 2008. www.nichd.nih.gov.

- According to the Down Syndrome Research and Treatment Foundation, researchers suspect that **only a small number of genes** significantly affect cognition.

- Researchers have found no evidence to support the theory that Down syndrome may be caused by **behavioral or environmental factors**.

# What Are the Ethical Issues of Down Syndrome?

**❝In my opinion, the moral thing for older mothers to do is to have amniocentesis . . . test whether placental cells have a third chromosome #21, and abort the fetus if it does.❞**

—Albert Harris, quoted in Samuel Spies, "Abortion Remark Angers Students."

**❝When I hear about people who have aborted such a child because they didn't want him to have to 'live a life like that,' I am incredulous. . . . What a travesty. What arrogance. What right do we have to destroy that little person because he doesn't measure up to someone's standard?❞**

—Lori Scheck, "A Normal Life."

When Martha Beck was pregnant with her son Adam, she learned through an amniocentesis that he had Down syndrome. She admits that the news was shocking to her, but she decided to go ahead with the pregnancy; and in doing so, she went against the strong recommendation of her obstetrician. He warned that things would never be the same for her and her husband and said that she was throwing her life away. He also told her that having a baby with Down syndrome would ruin her 18-month-old daughter's life. Although Beck did not feel that it was morally wrong for a woman to have an abortion after a diagnosis of Down syndrome, she believed it was the wrong decision for her. She ignored the physician's advice and had the baby, and her life did indeed change—for the better, as she writes:

> The fears and disadvantages of having such a child hit like a hammer blow at the moment of diagnosis. The gifts that come with these exceptional people make themselves known more slowly and subtly, over months, years, and decades. But for me, and most other parents of children with Down syndrome I know, these gifts end up far outweighing any pain or disappointment we may suffer because of our children's disabilities.[28]

## The Prenatal Testing Controversy

For years, only women over the age of 35 were advised to get prenatal screening for Down syndrome because their risk was so much higher than younger women's. Since such a high percentage of Down syndrome fetuses are aborted, this sort of testing has long been a source of major controversy—and the debate became even more heated in January 2007. The American College of Obstetricians and Gynecologists (ACOG) announced that it had revised its recommendation for prenatal testing to include all pregnant women, regardless of their age. The ACOG's announcement infuriated right-to-life organizations, as well as advocacy groups and families with children who have Down syndrome. George Will shares his views: "The ACOG guidelines are formally neutral concerning what decisions parents should make on the basis of the information offered," he writes.

> But what is antiseptically called "screening" for Down syndrome is, much more often than not, a search-and-destroy mission. . . . Nothing—*nothing*—in the professional qualifications of obstetricians and gynecologists gives them standing to adopt policies that predictably will have, and seem intended to have, the effect of increasing abortions in the service of an especially repulsive manifestation of today's entitlement mentality—every parent's "right" to a perfect baby.[29]

In spite of the ACOG's recommendation, many parents choose not to have prenatal tests. This was the decision made by Amy Julia Becker, the mother of a little girl with Down syndrome. When Becker was pregnant with her second child, a colleague said to her, "I assume you've done all the screening on this one to find out, if, you know, . . ."[30] Becker tried to explain why she was not going to have prenatal tests, saying that she was uncomfortable with the testing in general and that she was not particularly concerned about having another child with Down syndrome. The woman made it clear that she could not understand why Becker would make such a choice. Another expectant mother who opted not to have prenatal testing was Annette Reid, a woman from Canada who has a little girl with Down syndrome. Reid believes that doctors and social workers should be more careful in how they present information about Down syndrome to expectant mothers because the women may make an impulsive choice to abort and then regret it later. When Reid was pregnant, she decided that no matter what happened with her child, she would deal with it when the time came.

> **The American College of Obstetricians and Gynecologists (ACOG) announced that it had revised its recommendation for prenatal testing to include all pregnant women, regardless of their age.**

Contrary to what is often believed, not all pregnant women who have prenatal testing do so with the intention of getting an abortion if Down syndrome is diagnosed. Beth Spadaro's son was born with Down syndrome, and when he was three years old she became pregnant again. She decided to have an amniocentesis. "I just wanted to know," she says. "I love that little guy so much and I wouldn't change a thing about him, but if I was facing another challenging situation, I did not want to be surprised in the delivery room this time."[31] Spadaro ended up having a difficult, disturbing conversation with her physician's nurse, as she explains:

> When I called to set up the appointment for the amnio, the nurse said to me, in a very haughty tone, "Just so you

know, *this* doctor does *not* perform abortions." I was so shocked that I didn't know what to say. How dare she assume such a thing? And how dare she make such a hateful accusation toward me? That was never my intent, but it wasn't any of her business no matter what I decided. It was up to my husband and me, no one else. [32]

## When Test Results Are Wrong

One argument against prenatal testing is that the test results are not always correct. As the British Paediatric Neurology Association explains: "Just because you have an abnormality in a scan doesn't mean your baby will turn out abnormally."[33] After undergoing a magnetic resonance imaging (MRI) test, Becky and Kriss Kramer, a couple from the United Kingdom, were told that their unborn baby had multiple birth defects and would likely die shortly after birth. Doctors strongly urged the Kramers to terminate the pregnancy just a few weeks before the due date. They ignored the physicians' advice, and on October 1, 2007, Becky Kramer gave birth to a healthy baby boy whom she and her husband named Brandon. By the time Brandon was six months old, he was still in perfect health, was teething, and was attempting to walk. His mother later said that she felt a horrible sense of guilt whenever she thought that she might have taken the doctors' advice and aborted her son, and she wondered how many other babies had been inaccurately diagnosed when they were actually healthy.

> " Contrary to what is often believed, not all pregnant women who have prenatal testing do so with the intention of getting an abortion if Down syndrome is diagnosed. "

## Perfected Prenatal Testing?

One of the risks of many prenatal tests, including amniocentesis, is that they are invasive and thereby increase the risk of miscarriage. Also, such tests are not effective if they are performed too early in the pregnancy;

by the time abnormalities in the fetus are detected, the mother may be 5 or 6 months along. In June 2008 researchers in Hong Kong announced that they had developed a noninvasive test with at least a 90 percent accuracy rate for diagnosing Down syndrome that can be performed much earlier than other tests, as early as 7 weeks. It is a simple blood test that measures the way in which small amounts of fetal DNA and other chemicals cross the placenta to circulate in the mother's blood, and it can detect whether an extra copy of chromosome 21 is present. The new test is still in the trial stages; if all the trials conclude successfully, it could be available in 3 to 5 years.

> " Prenatal testing does not necessarily reveal the extent of birth defects, nor is there any way for physicians to know how severe a baby's mental retardation will be. "

People who are enthusiastic about the blood test argue that it will allow women who choose to have an abortion to make the decision earlier. Mothers who decide to go ahead with the pregnancy also benefit because they will have more time to prepare themselves for raising a child with disabilities. Those who are against the test say that it further increases the likelihood that babies with Down syndrome will be aborted, which they believe is unconscionable. Eunice Kennedy Shriver writes: "Prenatal testing by those with an intention to abort 'imperfect' human beings is a step backward. Science continues to identify causes of human imperfection. Where will it stop? Who will decide which characteristics are allowed and which are not?"[34]

## Quality of Life

Many people who decide to terminate a pregnancy after receiving a diagnosis of Down syndrome say that they are doing it for the sake of the child. Prenatal testing does not necessarily reveal the extent of birth defects, nor is there any way for physicians to know how severe a baby's mental retardation will be. When Maria Eftimiades' amniocentesis showed that her baby had Down syndrome, she feared for the child's future, as she explains: "To know now that our son would be retarded, perhaps profoundly, gives us the choice of not continuing the pregnancy. We don't want a life like that for our child, and the added worry that we wouldn't be around long enough to care for him throughout his life."[35] Eftimiades and the baby's father mutually decided that she would get an abortion. Although she grieved after the procedure was over and mourned the son she would never have, she was convinced that she made the right decision for her and her partner as well as for the child.

Martha Beck was also plagued with doubts and uncertainty when she found out that the baby she was carrying had Down syndrome. She was frightened that Adam would be rejected by a society that values perfection and superior intellect, and she was haunted by fears that her son would have a miserable life. These doubts were fueled by her obstetrician's negative comments, as she explains: "The most upsetting thing my ob-gyn doctor said as he tried to talk me into a therapeutic abortion was, 'You know this child will never be happy.' He compared Adam to a malignant tumor, a cellular accident that, left to grow, would lead to untold misery."[36] This was far from what actually happened, however. Beck says that Adam's life is "one of the happiest lives I've ever witnessed."[37] She adds that even though people with Down syndrome are all unique and different from each other, and have the same ups and downs in their lives as those who do not have the disorder, they appear to be more clear-sighted in one important way. "Instead of being diverted into chasing self-esteem in the form of honors, power, wealth, and competition," she writes,

> **" Prenatal testing allows expectant parents to learn in advance whether their unborn child has the disorder, and an estimated 90 percent of those who receive a positive diagnosis choose to have an abortion. "**

> they tend to remain focused on one primary criterion—love. When people have near-death experiences, they tend to react by putting love at the center of their lives.

The years they may have spent chasing happiness through conquest or acquisitiveness come to seem meaningless in comparison to the time they spent with the people and activities they most love. Adam, like other people with Down syndrome I know, never loses this perspective.[38]

Chris Burke is the epitome of someone with Down syndrome who lives life to its fullest. When Burke was born in 1965, doctors advised his parents to put him in an institution. Not only did his parents ignore the advice, they vowed to take their son home and treat him exactly the same as they did their other children. Throughout his childhood they encouraged him to think of his disorder as "Up syndrome." While he was growing up, Burke always dreamed of becoming an actor in Hollywood. "I didn't know how I would get there," he writes, "but I knew I was going to keep trying to make it come true."[39] In 1989 he got his wish when he landed the role of Corky Thatcher, a character with Down syndrome, in the television series *Life Goes On*. He continued with the series until 1993 and later founded and was lead singer for the musical group Chris Burke Band. Today, Burke is a well-known advocate for people with disabilities and is a goodwill ambassador for the National Down Syndrome Society. "The sky's the limit! Remember that!" he advises others who have Down syndrome. "Never give up. I'm trying my best and hardest to do everything I set out to do and you should too."[40]

## The Controversy Continues

The issue of Down syndrome is fraught with ethical considerations. Prenatal testing allows expectant parents to learn in advance whether their unborn child has the disorder, and an estimated 90 percent of those who receive a positive diagnosis choose to have an abortion. Others opt to continue with the pregnancy, believing that every life is worth saving regardless of their child having a disability. Will improved prenatal tests increase the number of Down syndrome babies who are aborted? Or will education and awareness about these children's potential motivate more parents to accept babies who have the disorder? No one knows. But Chris Burke and others like him hope to change the perception of Down syndrome so people focus on their abilities rather than their *dis*abilities.

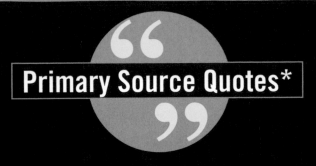

# Primary Source Quotes*

# What Are the Ethical Issues of Down Syndrome?

**"As a graduate student studying genetic disease, I hope that parents will harness the potential of widespread genetic testing (of both adults hoping to conceive and of fetuses) to eradicate a spectrum of painful and debilitating diseases."**

—William Motley, "To Raise a Down Syndrome Child," letter to the editor, *New York Times*, May 11, 2007. www.nytimes.com.

Motley is from Oxford, England, and is a doctoral candidate in genetics in a partnership program between the University of Oxford and the National Institutes of Health.

**"Now that medical science has enabled us to get a peek at an unborn person's genetic makeup, who decides who is entitled to an existence and who is not? Who determines whose life will have sufficient quality as to justify being born, and whose life should be snuffed out before they see the light of day?"**

—Tanya Holland, "Prof Wrong: Having Down Syndrome Doesn't Devalue a Person's Life," *Daily Advance*, March 11, 2008. www.dailyadvance.com.

Holland, a columnist for the *Daily Advance*, has a son with Down syndrome.

Bracketed quotes indicate conflicting positions.

* Editor's Note: While the definition of a primary source can be narrowly or broadly defined, for the purposes of Compact Research, a primary source consists of: 1) results of original research presented by an organization or researcher; 2) eyewitness accounts of events, personal experience, or work experience; 3) first-person editorials offering pundits' opinions; 4) government officials presenting political plans and/or policies; 5) representatives of organizations presenting testimony or policy.

Primary Source Quotes

66 People often say to us: 'How brave you are to have a child with Down Syndrome.' But it's not a question of courage: the dignity of each child is more important than its characteristics. 99

—Anna Oromi, "The Gift of a Child with Down Syndrome," Opus Dei, January 9, 2007. www.opusdei.us.

Oromi is a woman from Spain whose son Marc has Down syndrome.

66 Chromosomal abnormalities such as Down syndrome can often be diagnosed before birth by analyzing cells in the amniotic fluid or from the placenta. 99

—Children's Hospital Boston, "My Child Has Down Syndrome," 2007. www.childrenshospital.org.

Children's Hospital Boston is the primary pediatric teaching hospital of Harvard Medical School.

66 As science extends our capabilities to detect more and more conditions in the womb, as it inevitably will, I can't help asking if perhaps we should pause to ask if knowledge is always power. Should we have the right to determine who does and who doesn't get to inhabit the world? 99

—Rebecca Atkinson, "My Baby, Right or Wrong," *Guardian*, March 10, 2008. www.guardian.co.uk.

Atkinson, who suffers from a rare genetic disorder known as Usher syndrome, chose not to have prenatal testing for Down syndrome when she was pregnant.

66 When I look at my daughter and I think that there are people out there who think that she shouldn't have been born, how could you say she shouldn't be here? I don't understand. I want someone to explain to me why a child like mine is less worthy than somebody else's child. 99

—Catherine Pedler, "QLD Researchers Claim Down Syndrome Breakthrough," ABC Radio Australia, December 14, 2003. www.abc.net.au.

Pedler, who lives in Queensland, Australia, has a daughter with Down syndrome.

66 **While I have no doubt there can be joys and victories in raising a mentally handicapped child, for me and for Mike, it's a painful journey that we believe is better not taken. To know now that our son would be retarded, perhaps profoundly, gives us the choice of not continuing the pregnancy.** 99

—Maria Eftimiades, "One Woman's Choice," *Washington Post*, November 15, 2005. www.washingtonpost.com.

Eftimiades is a national correspondent for *People* magazine who chose to have an abortion when she learned that her son had Down syndrome.

66 **We were angry that someone would even suggest we might want to 'get rid of' our child, as if he were broken. But having been through this, it is very easy for me to understand how parents could be intimidated, subtly or otherwise, into aborting their child.** 99

—Laura Echevarria, "My Experience with Prejudice Against Children with Down Syndrome," *National Right to Life News*, May 2005.

Echevarria is the former director of media relations for National Right to Life.

66 **Many children with Down syndrome never get the chance to shed their light on the world.** 99

—Sydney, "The Upside of Down Syndrome," *Student Voice*, PBS, February 26, 2008.

Sydney is a teenage girl from Fresno, California, whose brother has Down syndrome.

66 **The National Down Syndrome Society does not take a position on abortion, recognizing that abortion is legal in the United States and that our constituents represent diverse backgrounds and philosophies.** 99

—National Down Syndrome Society (NDSS), "Abortion," 2008. www1.ndss.org.

NDSS's mission is to benefit people with Down syndrome and their families through national leadership in education, research, and advocacy.

**❝Screening women before the second trimester allows those who might opt to terminate a pregnancy to make that decision when doctors say an abortion is safer and less traumatic.❞**

—Rob Stein, "Down Syndrome Now Detectable in 1st Trimester," *Washington Post*, November 10, 2005.
www.washingtonpost.com.

Stein is a national science reporter for the *Washington Post*.

**❝In ancient Greece, babies with disabilities were left out in the elements to die. We in America rely on pre-natal genetic testing to make our selections in private, but the effect on society is the same.❞**

—Patricia E. Bauer, "The Abortion Debate No One Wants to Have," *Washington Post*, October 18, 2005.
www.washingtonpost.com.

Bauer, whose daughter has Down syndrome, is a former bureau chief and reporter for the *Washington Post*.

**❝Adoption agencies report a high demand for children with Down syndrome. However, the abortion rate for fetuses diagnosed with Down syndrome tops ninety percent.❞**

—Caitrin Nicol, "At Home with Down Syndrome," *New Atlantis*, Spring 2008.

Nicol is assistant editor of the *New Atlantis*.

# What Are the Ethical
# Issues of Down Syndrome?

- In 2007 the American College of Obstetricians and Gynecologists recommended that all pregnant women undergo **prenatal screening**, regardless of age.

- Approximately **70 percent** of pregnant women choose to undergo prenatal testing for Down syndrome and other genetic disabilities.

- An estimated **90 to 95 percent** of Down syndrome cases diagnosed through prenatal testing result in abortion.

- A 2004 survey of 1,126 mothers who had children with Down syndrome found that more than **85 percent** learned of the diagnosis after the babies were born.

- Amniocentesis **prenatal screening** cannot be performed until the fourteenth to eighteenth week of pregnancy.

- The most accurate type of prenatal test is known as **percutaneous umbilical blood sampling**, which cannot be done until the eigthteenth week of pregnancy and carries the highest risk of miscarriage.

- Statistics show that a high number of married couples who have babies with Down syndrome get **divorced**.

# Prenatal Screening

Pregnant women who want to find out if a fetus is healthy can undergo various types of prenatal testing. These tests have a high degree of accuracy, but they are controversial because an estimated 90 percent of Down syndrome diagnoses result in abortion. This chart describes three of the most common prenatal screening methods.

| Type | Process | When Performed | Accuracy Rate | Risk of Miscarriage |
|------|---------|----------------|---------------|---------------------|
| Chorionic Villus Sampling (CVS) | A small sample of cells (called chorionic villi) is taken from the placenta where it attaches to the wall of the uterus. The villi, which have the same genes as the fetus, are tested for the presence of extra material on chromosome 21. | Ninth to eleventh week of pregnancy | 98 percent | 1–2 percent |
| Amniocentesis | The physician guides a needle through the abdomen to remove some amniotic fluid. Cells contained within the fluid are analyzed in a laboratory to determine whether the fetus has Down syndrome or other genetic abnormalities. | Fourteenth to eighteenth week of pregnancy | More than 99 percent | Less than 1 percent |
| Percutaneous Umbilical Blood Sampling | The physician inserts a thin needle through the abdomen and uterine wall into the umbilical cord, then extracts a small sample of fetal blood. The blood is analyzed in the laboratory to detect the presence of extra material on chromosome 21. | Eighteenth to twenty-second week of pregnancy | The most accurate of all tests, and is used to confirm the results of CVS or amniocentesis | The highest risk of prenatal tests; mis-carriage occurs 1 to 2 times out of every 100 procedures. |

Sources: National Institute of Child Health and Human Development, "Facts About Down Syndrome," August 15, 2008. www.nichd.nih.gov; Web MD, "Prenatal Tests," September 22, 2007. www.webmed.com; American Pregnancy Association, "Percutaneous Umbilical Blood Sampling (PUBS): Also Known as Cordocentesis, Fetal Blood Sampling, and Umbilical Vein Sampling," September 2003. www.americanpregnancy.org.

## Americans' Views on Abortion

Although many expectant mothers opt not to have prenatal testing, an estimated 90 percent who do, and who receive a Down syndrome diagnosis, choose to terminate the pregnancy. From August 2007 to February 2008 the Ethics and Public Policy Center conducted a national survey of 1,003 American adults to gauge their views on abortion following prenatal screening. As this chart shows, their responses indicated that they were strongly against abortion unless the fetus was not expected to survive very long after birth.

*"New in-utero testing technologies are allowing parents to know in advance some of the genetic characteristics of their developing child fairly soon after conception, such as its sex or if it has any medical conditions or genetic diseases such as Down syndrome. In some cases, parents may choose to terminate or abort a pregnancy after learning the results of these tests. In which, if any, of the following circumstances do you believe parents should be legally allowed to terminate the pregnancy?"*

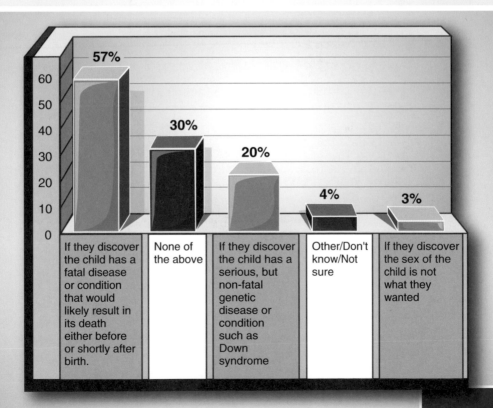

*Note: Survey totals more than 100 percent because respondents were allowed to give multiple answers to questions.*

Source: Yuval Levin, "Public Opinion and the Embryo Debates," *New Atlantis*, Spring 2008. www.thenewatlantis.com.

# Lack of Physician Support

Even though the potential for children born with Down syndrome has markedly improved in recent years, physicians still do not often know how to convey the diagnosis to parents without sounding negative. According to researcher Brian Skotko, many mothers who receive the diagnosis after the baby is born report fear and anxiety after learning of the disorder, and do not consider the overall experience to be positive. This graph shows how they responded to a survey published by Skotko in the January 2005 issue of *Pediatrics*.

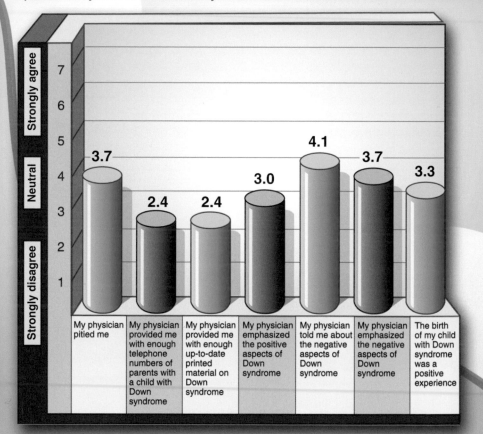

Source: Brian Skotko, "Mothers of Children with Down Syndrome Reflect on Their Postnatal Support," *Pediatrics*, January 2005. http://pediatrics.aappublications.org.

- Researchers have developed and are testing prenatal blood tests that are noninvasive and result in a **high degree of accuracy** at predicting Down syndrome.

- According to Harvard Medical School researcher Brian Skotko, many physicians admit that they have **little or no knowledge** of how to deliver the Down syndrome diagnosis to parents in a sensitive manner.

- In a 2003 survey of **28 ethics committees** in the United Kingdom, **95 percent** of respondents were in favor of prenatal screening for treatment of a life-threatening condition, while only **14 percent** were in favor of the screening if the diagnosis of Down syndrome would potentially lead to abortion.

# Will Science Someday Prevent Down Syndrome?

> **"Although individuals with DS currently still face a spectrum of obstacles, such as mental retardation, a growing amount of research may help further lighten their burden in the future."**
>
> —Society for Neuroscience, "Down Syndrome."

> **"I just hope there will always be a place in our society for children with Down syndrome."**
>
> —Sheila Hebein, quoted in Heather Sells, "The Blessing of a Down Syndrome Child."

O f all the scientists who have studied Down syndrome throughout history, no one was more passionate about his research than Jerome Lejeune. After he confirmed that the disorder was caused by extra genetic material on chromosome 21, Lejeune devoted the rest of his life to studying Down syndrome, and he was absolutely convinced that a cure would be found. His daughter Clara wrote about this in her memoir *Life Is a Blessing*, in which she stated that her father "believed it would take less work to cure Down syndrome than to travel to the moon."[41] Although Lejeune died before he could accomplish his goal, scientists continue to pursue research in the hope of learning why chromosomal abnormalities occur. If they are successful, they may someday be able to prevent or cure Down syndrome.

# Long-Range Research Plan

In January 2008 the National Institutes of Health (NIH) announced that it had embarked on an aggressive, 10-year research project that would focus on Down syndrome. The project came about after the NIH's National Institute of Child Health and Human Development (NICHD) formed a working group of NIH scientists. Through a series of public forums with families of children with Down syndrome, as well as major advocacy organizations, the group developed its long-range plan. The overall goal, according to the group, is "to build upon ongoing NIH-supported research relating to Down syndrome to reflect the changing lives of individuals and families affected, and to take advantage of emerging scientific opportunities."[42] One major focus of the plan is on increased research to study the medical, cognitive, and behavioral conditions that occur in people with Down syndrome, including accompanying diseases such as leukemia, heart disease, seizures, and stomach disorders, as well as mental health impairments. Another focus is on whether aging has a greater impact on mental capabilities in people with Down syndrome than in those who do not have the disorder. That knowledge could help scientists understand why such a large number of adults with Down syndrome suffer from Alzheimer's disease.

An integral part of the plan is a summary of the vast research efforts that are currently underway by the various NIH institutes. For instance, scientists at the NICHD are studying the role that the age of a mother's egg plays in the development of Down syndrome, while others

> " Although Lejeune died before he could accomplish his goal, scientists continue to pursue research in the hope of learning why chromosomal abnormalities occur. "

are researching specific genes and gene groups that may affect the onset of the disorder. The NIH's National Heart, Lung, and Blood Institute is supporting studies that analyze the genes that are believed to contribute to heart defects in children born with Down syndrome. The National Institute of Mental Health is studying the frequency and possible treatment of conditions such as autism, obsessive-compulsive disorder, depression, and psychosis in people with Down syndrome. The National Cancer Institute is studying various types of leukemia that typically affect children with the disorder, and the National Institute of Neurological Disorders and Stroke is investigating the various ways in which Down syndrome affects the brain.

## Cognitive Studies

In an effort to learn more about how Down syndrome causes learning disabilities, scientists at Stanford University have been performing experiments with laboratory mice. In 2006 they announced the discovery of one gene on chromosome 21 that could be connected with cognitive deficiencies in people with Down syndrome. The mice were genetically engineered to have the same chromosomal abnormalities that cause the disorder in humans. Some of the mice were bred to have an extra amount of a gene called App, which instructs the body to make a sticky protein known as beta-amyloid. Scientists know that when too much beta-amyloid builds up in the brain, it interferes with communication between neurons (brain cells). As a result, certain neurons that are essential for memory and learning wither and die. In their experiments the researchers found that the more App was present in the mice's bodies, the more neuron communication was hindered. They also observed that in mice that were bred to have extra chromosomal 21 material but not extra App, less brain damage occurred than in the mice with the excess App gene.

> " In August 2007 researchers at the University of Colorado at Denver announced that they may have found a method of reversing the learning impairments that are often associated with Down syndrome. "

This research is considered important because it could potentially lead to a treatment that targets just one gene, rather than having to correct the adverse effects of an entire chromosome, which is extremely challenging. William Mobley, lead author of the Stanford study, explains: "Some people think, 'My God, you'll never figure it out, you have to get rid of the whole chromosome. But it's really possible that beginning with a specific abnormality, you can chase it down—if not to one gene only, then to one gene that plays a major role. . . . Because you can do that, now you can think about therapies, which you couldn't really do before."[43]

## Potential Drug Treatments

In August 2007 researchers at the University of Colorado at Denver announced that they may have found a method of reversing the learning impairments that are often associated with Down syndrome. Their research involved testing the effectiveness of an FDA-approved drug known as memantine, which is normally used to treat patients with Alzheimer's disease. Mice that were bred to have Down syndrome, as well as a group of "control" mice without the disorder, were put in a chamber where they were exposed to a brief, mild electric shock that was designed to produce an unpleasant feeling without harming the creatures. The control mice showed fear and "froze up" when they were returned to the chamber 24 hours later, while the mice with Down syndrome could not recall the experience; they entered the chamber willingly and walked around without any sign of fear. The researchers then injected the Down syndrome mice with melantine at several different intervals, and when they were put back in the chamber they displayed the same fearful behavior as the control mice. In a paper that described the experiment, the scientists noted that this was "the first instance in which acute injection of a drug agent has improved the behavioral performance of Down syndrome in learning and memory."[44] In the future, such research could potentially lead to drug therapies that correct cognitive deficiencies and learning disabilities in people with Down syndrome.

## The Down Syndrome/Leukemia Connection

It has long been known that children with Down syndrome are at least 10 times more likely to develop leukemia than those who do not have the disorder. For years scientists have speculated that the extra genetic material on chromosome 21 was somehow responsible for this connection, but they did not know how or why this occurred. In December 2007 researchers from Tel Aviv University in Israel announced that they may have solved this puzzle. The research team, which was led by physician Shai Izraeli, analyzed blood samples from more than 8,000 children with acute lymphoblastic leukemia (ALL). They found that nearly one-fifth of the children who also had Down syndrome had a mutation on a gene known as Janus kinase 2 (JAK2), which could indicate that gene mutation is responsible for the increased risk of leukemia among children with the disorder. According to Izraeli, the researchers suspect that the extra genetic material on chromosome 21 gives a "survival advantage" to cells carrying the JAK2 mutation, meaning that cancerous cells are able to grow and thrive. He adds that scientists are currently working toward developing JAK2 inhibitors that could speed drug development for people with ALL and Down syndrome, as well as continuing to study the role that other genes might play.

## An Alternative Approach

Scientists have made excellent strides in their quest to better understand Down syndrome, and this has resulted in lifesaving treatment for health disorders, as well as more effective therapies, better educational opportunities, and overall improved quality of life. As research continues to progress, there may come a time when Down syndrome can be prevented or corrected in a child that is still in the womb—but not everyone is enthusiastic about that possibility. Many parents of children with Down syndrome believe that it is something to be celebrated rather than eliminated. Wesley J. Smith, a senior fellow at the Discovery Institute and the parent of a son with Down syndrome, shares his views: "I am here to tell you that Down's syndrome is not an insupportable horror for either the sufferer or the parents. I'll go further: human beings are not better off without Down's syndrome."[45]

> " It has long been known that children with Down syndrome are at least 10 times more likely to develop leukemia than those who do not have the disorder. "

Surveys have shown that numerous physicians still discourage expectant parents from going ahead with a pregnancy when Down syndrome has been diagnosed through prenatal testing. Many parents also report that after the baby's birth, health care professionals were not sensitive or supportive, nor did they help connect the parents with other families who have experience in dealing with the disorder. To remedy this situation, people throughout the country have formed a grassroots movement that seeks to educate expectant parents on what it is really like to raise a child with Down syndrome. They want these parents to understand that Down syndrome children can bring joy to their lives that they could not possibly foresee until they experience it for themselves. Group members are also motivated by the fear that expanded and improved prenatal testing will sharply reduce the number of children

> **Surveys have shown that numerous physicians still discourage expectant parents from going ahead with a pregnancy when Down syndrome has been diagnosed through prenatal testing.**

who are born with Down syndrome, which they believe would be tragic. One such parent is Nancy Iannone who lives in Turnersville, New Jersey. "For me, it's just faces disappearing," she says. "It isn't about abortion politics or religion, it's a pure ethical question."[46]

Although the advocacy movement is still in its infancy, it is growing, and members are starting to make themselves heard. Throughout the country parents of Down syndrome children are scheduling meetings with their local obstetricians to explain their group's purpose, and they are working to convince health care professionals to pass along information, including telephone numbers of group members, at the same time that they give prenatal test results to expectant parents. According to members of the movement, their goal is not to force their viewpoints on anyone, nor is it to pressure parents into parenting a child with disabilities. Rather, they are convinced that if more people were aware of the positive aspects of raising a Down syndrome child, as well as the massive difference that early intervention can make in a child's life, they might have second thoughts about aborting their baby.

In support of this grassroots movement, two U.S. senators proposed a piece of legislation in 2005 called the Prenatally Diagnosed Condition Awareness Act. The act was designed to ensure that prospective parents of babies with Down syndrome and other disabilities receive accurate, up-to-date information about life expectancy, intellectual and functional development, and prenatal and postnatal treatment options for their child. Those who support the legislation believe that it will help parents make a more informed decision after receiving a positive diagnosis from prenatal tests. In spite of overwhelming support from Down syndrome advocacy groups and parents, Congress did not pass the bill, and it was reintroduced for another vote in July 2007. As of August 2008 its status was still pending, although people who are in favor of it vow to keep fighting until it is finally passed and signed into law.

## An Uncertain Future

Historically, whenever scientists have developed a treatment or cure for a deadly disease, society has breathed a collective sigh of relief. Many diseases and disorders that formerly claimed the lives of nearly everyone who was afflicted are now, because of scientific progress, no longer a threat. Even the most serious diseases such as cancer, heart disease, diabetes, and epilepsy, among others, are treatable, and many people who suffer from them go on to live long lives. Although Down syndrome cannot be cured, and it cannot be corrected before birth, people who are born with it live longer, healthier, more fulfilling lives than ever before. Someday research may progress to the point where Down syndrome can be obliterated, and no one will ever have the disorder again. But is that a step in the right direction for science? Would the world really be a better place if no one had Down syndrome? Those are emotion-charged questions that have no easy answers—and no doubt the issue will be mired in controversy for many years to come.

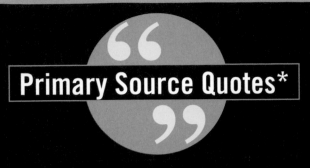

# Primary Source Quotes*

## Will Research Someday Prevent Down Syndrome?

66 Research on Down syndrome is making great strides in identifying the genes on chromosome 21 that cause the characteristics of Down syndrome. Scientists now feel strongly that it will be possible to improve, correct or prevent many of the problems associated with Down syndrome in the future. 99

—National Down Syndrome Society (NDSS), "Down Syndrome Myths & Truths," 2008. www1.ndss.org.

NDSS's mission is to benefit people with Down syndrome and their families through national leadership in education, research, and advocacy.

66 At the current rate, we will eventually exterminate children with Down from society. And the world will miss out on the opportunity to experience these wonderful and giving members of our communities. 99

—Valerie Karr, "Targeting the Womb, Down Syndrome, Disabilities," *Newsday*, July 7, 2008. www.newsday.com.

Karr is a PhD candidate at Columbia University who studies international perspectives on the rights of people with disabilities.

* Editor's Note: While the definition of a primary source can be narrowly or broadly defined, for the purposes of Compact Research, a primary source consists of: 1) results of original research presented by an organization or researcher; 2) eyewitness accounts of events, personal experience, or work experience; 3) first-person editorials offering pundits' opinions; 4) government officials presenting political plans and/or policies; 5) representatives of organizations presenting testimony or policy.

**❝I am against society imposing rules on individuals for how they want to use genetic knowledge. Just let people decide what they want to do.❞**

—James Watson, quoted in Tim Radford, "DNA Pioneer Urges Gene Free-for-All," *Guardian*, April 9, 2003. www.guardian.co.uk.

Watson is one of two scientists who discovered the double helix structure of DNA.

**❝I just read a long article about genetic engineering. . . . Because of this, we will eventually be able to find the genes that cause 'abnormalities' and eliminate, alter, and treat those genes so that 'abnormality' no longer appears in our society. Frankly, this scares the dickens out of me.❞**

—Donald C. Bakely, *Down Syndrome: One Family's Journey.* Cambridge, MA: Brookline Books, 2002.

Bakely, who has a daughter with Down syndrome, is an author and an advocate on behalf of people with disabilities as well as those who live in poverty.

**❝Advances in science always build on the work of the past, and today, we are positioned for a pace of progress that will be unlike anything ever dreamed of before.❞**

—Wayne Silverman, "Of Mice and Men," *Exceptional Parent*, July 2007.

Silverman is director of intellectual disabilities research at the Kennedy Krieger Institute in Baltimore, Maryland.

**❝A new generation of people with Down syndrome are living longer, finishing school, getting jobs and now—with a little help—beginning to marry.❞**

—Claudia Wallis, "A Very Special Wedding," *Time*, July 24, 2006.

Wallis is editor-at-large for *Time* magazine.

66 There are no inherent boundaries limiting the progress of a child with Down syndrome. Without a doubt,
they can progress at a much greater rate than is currently believed possible. 99

—Jenny Marrs, "John and the Art of Learning," National Association for Child Development, 2005. http://nacd.org.

Marrs is the mother of a son who has Down syndrome.

66 There's no medical cure for this condition. But increased understanding of Down syndrome and early
interventions make a big difference in the lives of both
children and adults with Down syndrome. 99

—Mayo Clinic, "Children's Health: Down Syndrome," April 6, 2007.

Mayo Clinic is a world-renowned medical facility that is dedicated to the diagnosis and treatment of virtually every type of illness.

66 The outlook for individuals with Down syndrome is far
brighter than it once was. Most of the health problems
associated with Down syndrome can be treated. 99

—March of Dimes, "Down Syndrome," March 2007. www.marchofdimes.com.

The March of Dimes is dedicated to improving the health of babies by preventing
birth defects, premature birth, and infant mortality.

**66** Perhaps one day Down syndrome will be considered a condition with which you can conceive. Can imagine. Can live. And not an experience to be avoided at all costs. **99**

—Fiona Place, "Amniocentesis and Motherhood: How Prenatal Testing Shapes Our Cultural Understandings of Pregnancy and Disability," *M/C Journal*, 2008. http://homepage.mac.com.

Place, an author from Australia, is the mother of a young boy who has Down syndrome.

**66** If Ned is to thrive in his world to come, he must be able to function with adults who don't particularly care whether he thrives or dies. **99**

—Greg Palmer, *Adventures in the Mainstream*. Bethesda, MD: Woodbine House, 2005.

Palmer is a writer and documentary producer whose son Ned has Down syndrome.

# Will Research Someday Prevent Down Syndrome?

- Presently, Down syndrome cannot be prevented, nor can the chromosomal abnormalities that cause it be **cured before a child is born**.

- According to the Down Syndrome Research and Treatment Foundation, scientists are extremely interested in studying the **hippocampus**, the area of the human brain that is essential for learning and memory.

- Much current research focuses on the underlying genetic and biological causes of **brain abnormalities** in children with Down syndrome.

- Mice are the preferred animals for studying Down syndrome because the mouse chromosome 16 **is strikingly similar** in structure to the human chromosome 21.

- Researchers in the United Kingdom have developed a **mouse model** that has a copy of the entire human chromosome 21.

- Scientists have found that the gene for a harmful protein that causes Alzheimer's disease is contained on **chromosome 21**; this knowledge could help explain why nearly all people with Down syndrome develop Alzheimer's.

- Because animal models have many limitations, researchers are searching for **human volunteers** to participate in clinical trials.

## Increased Life Expectancy

In the early twentieth century, children who were born with Down syndrome usually died very young. Today, most of the health problems associated with Down syndrome can be treated, so people are living much longer than in the past.

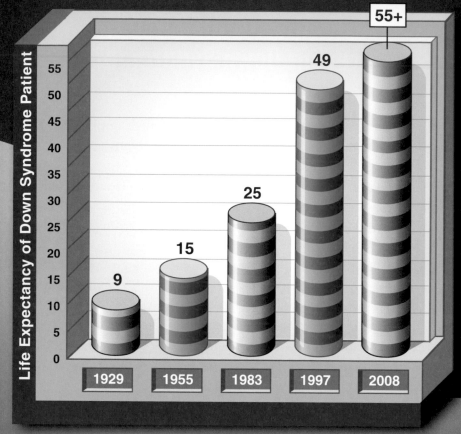

Sources: Q. Yang et al., "Mortality Associated with Down's Syndrome in the USA from 1983 to 1997: a Population-Based Study," *Lancet*, March 23, 2002; Gretel C. Kovach, "Celebration Honors 'Son,' Parents' Perseverance," *Dallas Morning News*, February 18, 2006. www.dallasnews.com.

- In June 2007 researchers at the Stanford University School of Medicine and Lucile Packard Children's Hospital **identified a gene** that, when overexpressed, caused neurons responsible for attention and memory to shrivel and stop functioning normally.

# Funding for Down Syndrome Research

Scientists have made great strides in understanding what causes Down syndrome, and they are hopeful that future studies will result in prevention or a cure. Such research is expensive, however, and will not be possible without adequate funding from public and private sources. This graph shows how federal funding for Down syndrome research compares with that of some other diseases and disorders.

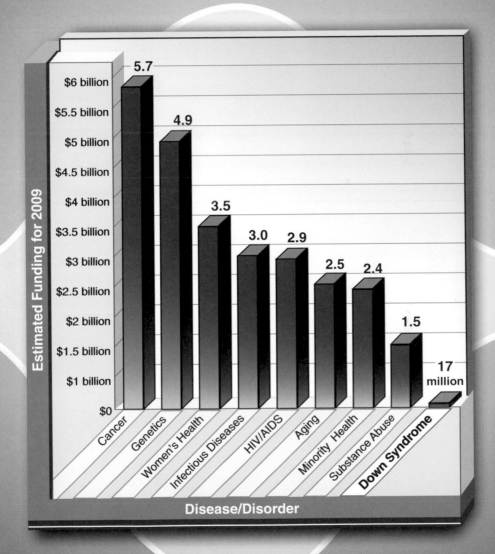

Source: Centers for Disease Control and Prevention, "National Estimates of and Racial and Ethnic Variations Among Selected Birth Defects," January 14, 2008. www.cdc.gov.

# Studying Down Syndrome with Stem Cells

Scientists have long believed that stem cells, which are the master cells capable of producing any type of cell in the body, have tremendous potential to treat and cure many diseases and disorders. In addition, stem cells can facilitate research. This illustration shows the process of creating stem cells from ordinary skin cells.

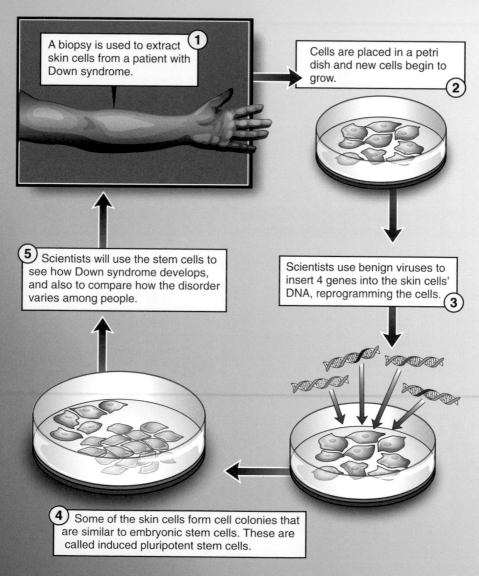

1. A biopsy is used to extract skin cells from a patient with Down syndrome.

2. Cells are placed in a petri dish and new cells begin to grow.

3. Scientists use benign viruses to insert 4 genes into the skin cells' DNA, reprogramming the cells.

4. Some of the skin cells form cell colonies that are similar to embryonic stem cells. These are called induced pluripotent stem cells.

5. Scientists will use the stem cells to see how Down syndrome develops, and also to compare how the disorder varies among people.

Sources: Maggie Fox, "Skin Cells Produce Library of Diseased Stem Cells," Reuters, August 7, 2008. www.reuters.com; Carolyn Y. Johnson, "Scientists Report a Breakthrough in Stem Cell Production," *Boston Globe*, August 1, 2008. www.boston.com.

- In February 2007 researchers at Stanford University School of Medicine and Lucile Packard Children's Hospital reported that a drug known as **PTZ** improved the learning and memory of lab mice with Down syndrome.

- In 2007 researchers learned that the same mutation on a gene known as JAK2 (found on chromosome 9) showed up in **20 percent** of people who had Down syndrome along with acute lymphoid leukemia, which suggests that the mutation increases the risk of someone developing the blood cancer.

- In May 2008 researchers from Cardiff University announced that children with Down syndrome who wore **bifocal lenses** for two years showed significant improvement in their ability to focus.

- In October 2007 researchers from the Children's Hospital of Philadelphia and the University of Pennsylvania School of Medicine found that **children with Down syndrome had higher levels of leptin**, a hormone linked to obesity, than their siblings who did not have the disorder, which could help explain why a high percentage of people with Down syndrome are overweight.

# Key People and Advocacy Groups

**Band of Angels Foundation:** An advocacy group, which was founded by a woman whose son has Down syndrome, that seeks to help children with the disorder reach their full potential.

**Chris Burke:** A man with Down syndrome who is a professional actor and musician, as well as an advocate on behalf of people with disabilities.

**John Langdon Down:** A British physician who studied and wrote about children with Down syndrome beginning in the mid-1800s, and for whom the disorder is named.

**Down Syndrome Research and Treatment Foundation (DSRTF):** An organization that supports biomedical research to accelerate the development of treatments to improve cognitive abilities in people with Down syndrome.

**Sandra Jensen:** A California woman with Down syndrome who generated national publicity when she fought for the right to have a heart and lung transplant in 1996, and became the first persen with the disorder to have such an operation.

**Jerome Lejeune:** A prominent French geneticist who confirmed that trisomy 21 is a genetic disorder caused by chromosomal abnormalities.

**March of Dimes:** An organization whose mission is to improve the health of babies by preventing birth defects, premature birth, and infant mortality.

**National Association for Down Syndrome:** An advocacy group whose mission is to avail all people with Down syndrome of opportunities to achieve their potential in all aspects of community life.

**National Down Syndrome Society:** An organization that seeks to benefit people with Down syndrome and their families through national leadership in education, research, and advocacy.

**National Institute of Child Health and Human Development (NICHD):** An organization that is dedicated to conducting and supporting research that will benefit the health of children, adults, families, and populations.

**Eunice Kennedy Shriver:** An advocate on behalf of those who have Down syndrome, Shriver is outspoken about her objection to Down syndrome babies being aborted.

**George Will:** A conservative columnist and commentator whose oldest son has Down syndrome.

# Chronology

**1865**
Austrian scientist Gregor Mendel publishes his laws of genetics and eventually becomes known as the Father of Genetics.

**1953**
Scientists James Watson and Francis Crick discover the double helix structure of DNA.

**1866**
British physician John Langdon Down provides the first description of the disorder that comes to be known as Down syndrome.

**1902**
American biologist Walter Sutton demonstrates that chromosomes exist in pairs that have similar structures.

1865       1900       1950

**1887**
Down publishes *On Some of the Mental Affections of Childhood and Youth*, in which he describes the startlingly similar physical features of patients with Down syndrome.

**1956**
Scientists Albert Levan and Joe-Hin Tijo publish their discovery that humans have 46 chromosomes.

**1920**
The average life expectancy for a child with Down syndrome is nine years.

**1882**
By staining cells with dyes, German biologist Walter Fleming discovers rod-shaped objects he calls "chromosomes."

**1958**
French geneticist Jerome Lejeune confirms that Down syndrome is caused by an extra chromosome 21, and he names the disorder trisomy 21.

**1975**
Congress passes the Education of All Handicapped Children Act, which mandates a free, appropriate public education for children with Down syndrome and other disabilities. The law is later renamed the Individuals with Disabilities Education Act.

**2008**
The average life expectancy for people with Down syndrome has risen to mid-fifties.

**1987**
A gene that causes Alzheimer's disease is found on chromosome 21.

**2005**
British scientists create the first laboratory mouse with the equivalent of Down syndrome.

1975        1985        1995        2005

**1983**
The average life expectancy for people with Down syndrome is 25 years.

**2007**
The American College of Obstetricians and Gynecologists expands its recommendation for prenatal testing to include all pregnant women, regardless of age.

**1979**
The National Down Syndrome Society is founded by Betsy Goodwin.

**1990**
Congress passes the Americans with Disabilities Act, which guarantees that people with disabilities cannot be discriminated against.

# Related Organizations

### American College of Obstetricians and Gynecologists (ACOG)

409 12th St. SW

PO Box 96920

Washington, DC 20090-6920

phone: (202) 638-5577

Web site: www.acog.org

ACOG, which has more than 50,000 members, serves as an advocate for quality health care for women. A variety of pamphlets, educational materials, and other publications relating to Down syndrome are available on its Web site.

### Band of Angels Foundation

3048 Charlwood Dr.

Rochester Hills, MI 48306

phone: (248) 377-9309 • fax: (248) 230-3146

Web site: www.bandofangels.com

Band of Angels seeks to help children who have Down syndrome reach their full potential, beginning with providing accurate and positive information about the syndrome at the time of diagnosis. Its Web site contains information about Down syndrome, an "Angel Gallery" with photos of children, and news articles.

### Down Syndrome Research Foundation and Resource Centre (DSRF)

3580 Slocan St.

Vancouver, BC V5M 3E8 Canada

phone: (604) 431-9694 • fax: (604) 431-9248

e-mail: dsrf@sfu.ca • Web site: www.dsrf.org

DSRF's mission is to help people with Down syndrome achieve their potential, lead independent and fulfilling lives, and participate fully in their communities. Its Web site offers news articles, a vast amount of information about Down syndrome, and research publications.

## Down Syndrome Research and Treatment Foundation (DSRTF)

755 Page Mill Rd., Suite A-200

Palo Alto, CA 94304-1005

phone: (650) 468-1668 • fax: (650) 851-7258

e-mail: dsrtf@dsrtf.org • Web site: www.dsrtf.org

The DSRTF supports biomedical research that will accelerate the development of treatments to improve cognition for people with Down syndrome. Information available on its Web site includes facts about Down syndrome, research findings, FAQs, and newsletters.

## March of Dimes

1275 Mamaroneck Ave.

White Plains, NY 10605

phone: (888) 663-4637

e-mail: info@marchofdimes.com • Web site: www.marchofdimes.com

March of Dimes's mission is to improve the health of babies by preventing birth defects, premature birth, and infant mortality. Its Web site offers information about chromosomal abnormalities, facts about birth defects, state graphs and maps, and a Down syndrome reference page.

## National Association for Down Syndrome (NADS)

PO Box 206

Wilmette, IL 60091

phone: (630) 325-9112

e-mail: info@nads.org • Web site: www.nads.org

The NADS offers information, support, and advocacy to achieve its mission of allowing all people with Down syndrome to have opportunities to achieve their potential in all aspects of community life. Its Web site offers Down syndrome facts, human interest stories, a discussion forum, book reviews, and the NADS newsletter.

### National Down Syndrome Congress (NDSC)

7000 Peachtree-Dunwoody Rd. NE, Bldg. 5, Suite 100

Atlanta, GA 30328-1662

phone: (770) 604-9500 • toll free: (800) 232-6372

Web site: www.ndsccenter.org

The NDSC provides information, advocacy, and support concerning all aspects of life for individuals with Down syndrome. Its annual report is available on the Web site, along with a *Governmental Affairs Newsline* publication, news stories, and resources for parents.

### National Down Syndrome Society (NDSS)

666 Broadway

New York, NY 10012

phone: (212) 460-9330 • toll-free: (800) 221-4602

Web site: www.ndss.org

The mission of the NDSS is to benefit people with Down syndrome and their families through national leadership in education, research, and advocacy. Its Web site offers news articles, fact sheets, and numerous downloadable brochures.

### National Institute of Child Health and Human Development (NICHD)

NICHD Clearinghouse

PO Box 3006

Rockville, MD 20847

phone: (800) 370-2943

Web site: www.nichd.nih.gov

The NICHD conducts and supports research on topics related to the health of children, adults, families, and populations. Its Web site's search engine produces numerous Down syndrome publications, fact sheets, and research papers.

## National Institutes of Health (NIH)

9000 Rockville Pike

Bethesda, MD 20892

phone: (301) 496-4000

e-mail: nihinfo@od.nih.gov • Web site: www.nih.gov

The NIH, the leading medical research organization in the United States, is the primary federal agency for conducting and supporting medical research. NIH scientists search for ways to improve human health as well as investigate the causes, treatments, and possible cures for diseases. Using the Web site's search engine produces a number of articles and fact sheets about Down syndrome.

# For Further Research

## Books

William I. Cohen, Lynn Nadel, and Myra E. Madnick, eds., *Down Syndrome: Visions for the 21st Century*. New York: Wiley-Liss, 2002.

Jennifer Graf Groneberg, *Road Map to Holland*. New York: New American Library, 2008.

Janice Credit Houska, *For the Love of Matthew*. Victoria, BC: Trafford, 2006.

Cynthia S. Kidder and Brian Skotko, *Common Threads: Celebrating Life with Down Syndrome*. Rochester Hills, MI: Band of Angels, 2001.

Jason Kingsley and Mitchell Levitz, *Count Us In: Growing Up with Down Syndrome*. Orlando, FL: Harcourt, 2007.

Dawn Laney, *Down Syndrome*. Detroit: Greenhaven, 2008.

Greg Palmer, *Adventures in the Mainstream*. Bethesda, MD: Woodbine House, 2005.

Siegfried M. Pueschel, *Adults with Down Syndrome*. Baltimore: Paul H. Brooks, 2006.

Joyce Sampson, *Down (Syndrome) but Not Out*. Enumclaw, WA: Winepress, 2007.

Kathryn Synard Soper, *Gifts: Mothers Reflect on How Children with Down Syndrome Enrich Their Lives*. Bethesda, MD: Woodbine House, 2007.

## Periodicals

Lori Berger, "An Unexpected Blessing," *Redbook*, June 2005.

Nina Burleigh, "On Her Own," *People Weekly*, October 16, 2006.

Laura Echevarria, "Not an 'Error' but Our Child," *National Right to Life News*, February 2006.

Tom Groneberg, "My Partner in Patience," *Best Life*, October 2007.

Sanjay Gupta, "Should Baby Be Scanned?" *Time*, February 5, 2007.

Mary Cleary Kiely, "Slow Learners," *U.S. Catholic*, August 2007.

Lizzie Martinez, "Enjoying My Daughter with Down Syndrome," *Mothering*, March/April 2005.

Sue Mayer, "Sam's Journey to 'Reach for the Stars,'" *Exceptional Parent*, February 2007.

Carol Midgley, "Disability Dolls: A Blessing for Kids, or Just a Sick Joke?" *Times* (London), June 25, 2008.

Caitrin Nicol, "At Home with Down Syndrome," *New Atlantis*, Spring 2008.

Melissa Riggio, "I Have Down Syndrome: Know Me Before You Judge Me," *National Geographic Kids*, December 2006.

Julie Scharper, "After High School, Her Time to Shine," *Baltimore Sun*, June 2, 2008.

Eunice Kennedy Shriver, "Prenatal Testing: Supporting Parents of Children with Down Syndrome," *America*, May 14, 2007.

Wayne Silverman, "Of Mice & Men," *Exceptional Parent*, July 2007.

Claudia Wallis, "The Down Dilemma: Is a Life with the Syndrome Worth Living?" *Time*, November 21, 2005.

## Internet Sources

Patricia E. Bauer, "If the Test Says Down Syndrome," *Washington Post*, November 16, 2007. www.washingtonpost.com/wp-dyn/content/article/2007/11/15/AR2007111502031.html.

Amy Julia Becker, "Down Syndrome Is a Part of Who My Daughter Is," *Philadelphia Inquirer*, July 20, 2008. www.philly.com/inquirer/currents/20080720_Down_syndrome_is_a_part_of_who_my_daughter_is.html.

Beverly Beckham, "An Extra Chromosome Isn't Awful," *Boston Globe*, November 20, 2005. www.boston.com/news/local/articles/2005/11/20/an_extra_chromosome_isnt_awful.

Maria Eftimiades, "One Woman's Choice," *Washington Post*, November

15, 2005. www.washingtonpost.com/wp-dyn/content/article/2005/11/11/AR2005111102212_pf.html.

Maggie Fox, "Down Syndrome Protein May Deter Cancer," *Boston Globe*, January 3, 2008. www.boston.com/news/nation/articles/2008/01/03/down_syndrome_protein_may_deter_cancer.

Valerie Karr, "Targeting the Womb, Down Syndrome, Disabilities," *Newsday*, July 7, 2008. www.newsday.com/news/opinion/ny-opxxx5755254jul07,0,5073863.story.

March of Dimes, "Down Syndrome," March 2007. www.marchofdimes.com/professionals/14332_1214.asp.

National Institutes of Health, "Research Plan on Down Syndrome," October 2007. www.nichd.nih.gov/publications/pubs/upload/NIH_Downsyndrome_plan.pdf.

Margaret Renkl, "Life with Anthony," *Parenting*, December 2007. www.parenting.com/article/Pregnancy/Development/Life-With-Anthony.

Sally Sara, "For People with Down Syndrome, Longer Life Has Complications," *New York Times*, June 1, 2008. www.nytimes.com/2008/06/01/nyregion/01down.html.

George F. Will, "Golly, What Did Jon Do?" *Newsweek*, January 29, 2007. www.newsweek.com/id/70159.

# Source Notes

## Overview

1. John Langdon Down, *On Some of the Mental Affections of Childhood and Youth*. London: J&A Churchill, 1887, pp. 7–8.
2. National Down Syndrome Society, "Down Syndrome," 2008. www1ndss. org.
3. Martha Beck, "The Gifts of Down Syndrome: Some Thoughts for New Parents," in William I. Cohen et al., eds., *Down Syndrome*. New York: Wiley-Liss, 2002, p. 141.
4. Andrea Lack, "Turning the Vision into Reality," in Cohen et al., eds., *Down Syndrome*, p. 442.
5. Quoted in Michael Amsel, "Her Family's Love Helps Woman with Down Syndrome Enjoy Life," *Asbury Park Press*, August 3, 2008. http://app.com.
6. H. Fisch et al., "The Influence of Paternal Age on Down Syndrome," *Journal of Urology*, June 2003. www.ncbi.nlm. nih.gov.
7. Fisch et al., "The Influence of Paternal Age on Down Syndrome."
8. Quoted in Laura Echevarria, "Not an 'Error' but Our Child," *National Right to Life News*, February 2006, p. 4.
9. National Down Syndrome Society, "Early Intervention & Down Syndrome," 2008. www1.ndss.org.
10. U.S. Office of Special Education Programs, "History: Twenty-Five Years of Progress in Educating Children with Disabilities Through IDEA," 2001. www.ed.gov.
11. ADA, "Americans with Disabilities Act of 1990." www.ada.gov.
12. Valerie Karr, "Targeting the Womb, Down Syndrome, Disabilities," *Newsday*, July 7, 2008. www.newsday.com.
13. Wayne Silverman, "Of Mice & Men," *Exceptional Parent*, July 2007, p. 106.
14. Elizabeth Schiltz, "Down Syndrome and the Pressure to Abort," ZENIT, March 9, 2006. www.zenit.org.

## What Is Down Syndrome?

15. George F. Will, "Golly, What Did Jon Do?" *Newsweek*, January 29, 2007. www.newsweek.com.
16. Susan Snashall, "Hearing Impairment & Down's Syndrome," St. George's University of London, *Learning About Intellectual Disabilities and Health*, 2002. www.intellectualdisability.info.
17. Quoted in About Down Syndrome, "Physical Therapy in Down Syndrome," 2006. www.about-down-syn drome.com.
18. Donald C. Bakely, *Down Syndrome: One Family's Journey*. Cambridge, MA: Brookline Books, 2002, pp. 63–64.
19. Bakely, *Down Syndrome: One Family's Journey*, pp. 228–29.
20. Joseph R. Carcione, ed., "Alzheimer's Disease: Understanding How Down Syndrome Increases Risk," WebMD, January 1, 2007. www.webmd.com.
21. Quoted in Sally Sara, "For People with Down Syndrome, Longer Life Has Complications," *New York Times*, June 1, 2008. www.nytimes.com.
22. Eunice Kennedy Shriver, "Prenatal Testing: Supporting Parents of Children with Down Syndrome," *America*, May 14, 2007, pp. 20–21.

## What Causes Down Syndrome?

23. National Human Genome Research Institute, "Chromosomes," May 19, 2008. www.genome.gov.
24. Christina Molin, "Should Have Played

the Lottery," *Prince Vince Meets the World*, June 15, 2006. http://christina molin.wordpress.com.

25. National Down Syndrome Society, "What Is Mosaicism?" 2008. www1. ndss.org.

26. National Institute of Child Health and Human Development, "Facts About Down Syndrome," August 18, 2006. www.nichd.nih.gov.

27. Quoted in Steve Quinn, "Alaska Governor Balances Newborn's Needs, Official Duties," *USA Today*, May 10, 2008. www.usatoday.com.

## What Are the Ethical Issues of Down Syndrome?

28. Beck, "The Gifts of Down Syndrome," p. 138.

29. Will, "Golly, What Did Jon Do?"

30. Quoted in Amy Julia Becker, "Down Syndrome Is a Part of Who My Daughter Is," *Philadelphia Inquirer*, July 20, 2008. www.philly.com.

31. Beth Spadaro, interview with author, August 1, 2008.

32. Spadaro, interview.

33. Quoted in Devon Williams, "Healthy Baby Born Despite Test," *Tulsa Beacon*, April 17, 2008. www.tulsabeacon. com.

34. Shriver, "Prenatal Testing: Supporting Parents of Children with Down Syndrome."

35. Maria Eftimiades, "One Woman's Choice," *Washington Post*, November 15, 2005. www.washingtonpost.com.

36. Beck, "The Gifts of Down Syndrome," p. 140.

37. Beck, "The Gifts of Down Syndrome," p. 141.

38. Beck, "The Gifts of Down Syndrome," p. 141.

39. Chris Burke, "Follow Your Dreams," in William I. Cohen et al., eds., *Down Syndrome*. New York: Wiley-Liss, 2002, p. 113.

40. Burke, "Follow Your Dreams," p. 114.

## Will Science Someday Prevent Down Syndrome?

41. Quoted in Leticia Velasquez, "Down, Not Out," *National Catholic Register*, July 6–12, 2008. www.ncregister. com/site/article/15354.

42. NIH Down Syndrome Working Group, "National Institutes of Health Research Plan on Down Syndrome," October 2007. www.nichd.nih.gov.

43. Quoted in Carey Goldberg, "Research Stirs Hope on Down Syndrome," *Boston Globe*, July 10, 2006. www.boston. com.

44. Quoted in University of Colorado at Denver, "New Research Uncovers Clue to Help Down Syndrome Patients Increase Learning Capacity," news release, August 20, 2007. www.uchsc. edu.

45. Wesley J. Smith, "Politically Correct Eugenics," *Weekly Standard*, March 31, 2008.

46. Quoted in Amy Harmon, "Prenatal Test Puts Down Syndrome in Hard Focus," *New York Times*, May 9, 2007. www.nytimes.com.

# List of Illustrations

# Index

# About the Author

Peggy J. Parks holds a bachelor of science degree from Aquinas College in Grand Rapids, Michigan, where she graduated magna cum laude. She is an author who has written more than 70 nonfiction educational books for children and young adults, as well as self-publishing her own cookbook called *Welcome Home: Recipes, Memories, and Traditions from the Heart*. Parks lives in Muskegon, Michigan, a town that she says inspires her writing because of its location on the shores of Lake Michigan.